I'M STILL KICKIN'

Overcoming the Impossible When You're Mad at the World

Brandon Mouw

IMAGINEWE
Publishers™

ImagineWe Publishers
New York - Florida South Carolina

Published by: ImagineWe, LLC
ImagineWe Publishers
247 Market Street, Suite 201
Lockport, NY 14094
United States
imaginewellc.com

© 2021 ImagineWe, LLC

ISBN: 978-1-946512-41-3
Library of Congress Control Number: 2021941002

First Edition

We are always looking for new authors ages five and up. For more information, please visit the website listed above. To shop our selection of books and merchandise you can visit: www.bookstore.imaginewellc.com

Contents

FOREWORD

Edmund Huang, M.D.

"The difference between a successful person and others is not a lack of strength, not a lack of knowledge, but rather a lack of will."

-Vince Lombardi, Associate Professor

Perseverance is a virtue. A person's limitations can often be overcome with enough determination and hard work. One can study harder, work more, sleep less. But, what do you do when your best efforts are not enough?

I met Brandon Mouw in June 2019 after he moved from Arizona back home to California. At the time, he was approximately six months removed from a pancreas transplant and was looking for a transplant physician in Los Angeles. The first line of my initial consultation note describes Brandon well. It states, "Mr. Mouw is a 34 year old male with a history of Type 1 Diabetes diagnosed at the age of 3. He had problems with hypoglycemic unawareness and was pronounced dead twice before. He therefore pursued pancreas transplant alone, but because insurance did not cover this kind of transplant, he paid out of pocket and had the procedure performed on 12/27/2018 at Mayo Arizona." Very few people encounter challenges of this nature in their lifetime, let alone by the age of 34. The Bible says that God "will not let you be tempted beyond what you can bear. But when you are tempted, He will also provide a way out so that you can endure it." (1 Corinthians 10:13) God chose Brandon, perhaps because He knew Brandon could handle it. Or, perhaps because he knew Brandon needed to endure these obstacles in order to grow from them.

From an early age, Brandon acquired the tenacity that would help him overcome increasingly larger obstacles later on. Relying on his own skills, Brandon was successful in almost everything because of his ability. A chronic illness, however, was something even Brandon could not control. Resourcefulness, perseverance, and talent alone were not enough to manage the vagaries of brittle Type 1 Diabetes and Brandon's life was spiraling out of control. Along the way, he discovered qualities exemplified in others that were equally as important as perseverance: trust, faithfulness, generosity, compassion, and love.

I'm Still Kickin': Overcoming the Impossible When You're Mad at the World is a story about managing and overcoming the cruelties of life. Life is not fair – nobody deserves to grow up diabetic or confront death at such a young age. We will never know why bad things seem to happen to some and not others. But, we can't stay angry at the world. Perhaps Vince Lombardi wasn't entirely accurate in highlighting will as the key to success. Overcoming life's obstacles isn't about strength, talent, or resolve – we need others and can't succeed on our own ability. Brandon's story is about finding the good in others, and in doing so, discovering the good things in life – even when you have every reason to be mad at the world.

CHAPTER 1

The Disorderly Kidney

L ife doesn't always work out the way you expect it. I learned this the hard way, after thinking I had figured it all out, through chronic illness, backstabbing betrayal, and the biggest surprise even I could ever imagine.

But first, let me take you back to a time I found happiness I didn't believe existed any longer.

I hadn't felt this sense of weightless joy since I was a little kid, helping my mom and dad on our egg ranch in California. Back on the ranch, there was always work to be done. I had a purpose. I had a job. I knew I was doing something meaningful by helping out the family business. But when all of that got taken away, I never thought I'd find purpose again.

Until now. Through trial and, well, I wouldn't say error. But I finally found something I loved: law school. I felt like every single thing I learned was valuable and could be applied to real life.

Nothing felt mindless and nothing felt like busywork.

I spent years finding my place in the world and in the blistering heat of Arizona in 2015, I knew I was on the right track. On one of those hot Wednesdays in June, I felt a twitch of pain in my back. I didn't think much of it at first. It could be the heat. It could be from carrying my law school textbooks to class. It could be from a sore muscle from a hike. It could be that I slept funny the night before.

Two days went by, but the pain remained. By Friday evening, it had grown worse. I touched the area tenderly with my left hand to find the source of the pain, but my skin didn't feel abnormal. Despite a lack of physical evidence on the outside, I knew this was something more serious than a sore muscle. It was too late for a doctor's appointment. *I can wait until Monday*, I thought. *I'll sleep it off.* I took a cool shower and crawled into bed. The pain was too uncomfortable. Stabbing. I rolled around trying to find a comfortable spot. *Maybe the pain was moving around from my back to the front of my left side?* Comfort kept eluding me.

Frustrated, I grabbed my phone and spent the next three hours looking up symptoms to make a self-diagnosis. It felt much worse than a muscle strain. The pain was getting worse, and I started to get concerned. *Sleep, Brandon. You can go to a doctor on Monday.*

Saturday there was no improvement, and I was determined to wait it out as long as possible to go to my trusted doctor first thing Monday morning. *Just one more day to go*, I told myself. I made it to Saturday night and tried once more to sleep it off. *"Ahhhhh!"* All of the sudden a burst of pain shot through my body, overtaking every muscle fiber. I fell to the floor when I jumped out of the bed, rolling back and forth. I gasped for air and clenched my jaw. The pain was like an elephant stepping on the left side of my back, crushing all my insides. It also felt like little perfectly sharpened knives were puncturing my abdomen, over and over and over. As I reached for my phone, it tumbled several feet away. I crawled toward it and tried to look up nearby urgent care centers but it was no use.

Nothing was open. I tried to pull myself off the floor back onto my bed. I felt weak, and my breathing was labored as I started to sweat. Around 3:00 a.m., I somehow catapulted out of bed and looked at my reflection in the mirror. I was sweating profusely, pale, nearly translucent, and trembling.

I grabbed my phone again and searched "hospital." About 15 minutes later, I was driving up to the hospital. I was relieved to find the triage line wasn't too long.

"Hi, my name is Brandon. I am a juvenile type 1 diabetic, and I have horrible pain going up and down my left side of my back. Something is not right," I said as my body continued to tremble.

I can't imagine what I looked like to someone on the outside. The nurse told me to sit down, and that they would take me back as quickly as they could. Ambulances started showing up. Someone was stabbed. Someone else had been in a car accident and I sat there looking like nothing was physically wrong. Less than five minutes later, they called me back. Everyone in the waiting room looked at me, possibly surprised I was called in before them. I dropped my eyes to the floor and quickly followed the nurse through the doorway. After a few initial questions, the nurse came in with needles and an IV, preparing to take my blood and administer medicine.

I held my breath. I hated hospitals. And I really hated having my blood drawn. I had not been a patient in a hospital since I was a little kid. I could still remember that horrifying evening when my parents took me to Loma Linda Children's Hospital.

I'm Still Kickin'

I was three years old when my parents noticed that I went from being an effervescent kid with abundant energy to being extremely lethargic. Concerned, my parents took me to Loma Linda Children's Hospital. Once we got there, a strange person picked me up and took me away from my parents in the waiting room. It happened so fast I didn't even get a chance to say goodbye. I watched the walls and doorways pass by as I was helplessly carried into a room down the hall. The stranger entered a cold and dark room and placed me on an icy metal table. There were no comfortable beds or plush animals to ease my discomfort. It was a bare metal table in a scary cold room. My three-year-old brain started to panic as I thought I had been kidnapped. Surely, my parents would come rescue me.

I wriggled on the table as a very large man held me down. I felt the cold table press into my back as my eyes darted back and forth, searching for clues to my predicament. A lady walked in and began to pop open bottles and needles and grabbed my arm. Suddenly, a sharp pain radiated from my arm as a needle pierced my skin. Blood began to flow out from the needle into a series of tubes. I was terrified. After what seemed like hours (but was probably about five or ten minutes), I was returned to my parents—a sobbing, scared mess. That one experience traumatized me for life and it came with a lifetime diagnosis of Juvenile Diabetes (Type 1 Diabetes).

*   *   *

Diabetes is a very real physical disease, and it comes with high and low blood sugars. There are different types of Diabetes: specifically Type 1 and Type 2. It is important to understand the difference in order to understand my story.

Type 1 Diabetes is rare and used to be called juvenile-onset Diabetes or insulin-dependent Diabetes. It is usually diagnosed during childhood. Type 1 Diabetes occurs when the pancreas cannot produce insulin because the body's immune system attacks and destroys insulin producing cells in the pancreas. There are no direct underlying causes or links as to why the body begins to attack the pancreas. A Type 1 Diabetic is reliant on insulin for the rest of their life. There is no prevention, reversal, or cure.

On the other hand, Type 2 Diabetes makes up more than 90% of diabetic diagnoses. It typically affects those who are older and is usually caused by lifestyle choices. People with Type 2 Diabetes still produce insulin, but do not make enough insulin for their body. In most cases, Type 2 Diabetes can be managed through diet, exercise, medication, and can even be reversed.

*   *   *

And now here I was back in the hospital, an adult, about to be pricked and prodded, again knowing I could handle the pain, but thinking back on that first blood draw. "Just a little pinch," the nurse said sympathetically as she inserted the needle into my skin. I had to look away. Within a few minutes, the morphine started coursing through my veins and the pain subsided. I felt much better as the doctors came in to poke and prod me. Next they transported me to radiology for an X-ray and then a CT scan.

Even though it was in the wee hours of the morning and something could seriously be wrong with me, I was relieved to be out of pain. Whatever it was, it was being handled. But, I wasn't sure what it was. Half an hour later, I had five or six doctors hovering over me, each one staring at me with confused and bewildered expressions. I felt like a specimen, or some scientific discovery in a petri dish.

"What's going on?" I asked them calmly. I wanted them to get straight to the point. While I did think it was strange there were so many people, I assumed they were different specialists. Growing up,

I always had a primary care or family doctor and an endocrinologist because of my diabetes.

"Brandon, how did you get here?" one of the physicians asked me. I didn't understand why my question was met with another question.

"I drove," I replied.

"How long have you had these symptoms?" another asked.

"I started having the pain on Wednesday. It got worse each day, but it was tolerable until tonight."

I scanned the room, pausing a few seconds to look each doctor in the eye. *What the hell is going on?*

"Your CT scan shows that your left kidney is the size of a football. You have two kidney stones about as big as your thumbnail lodged in the kidney, which is preventing urine from draining to the bladder and contributing to the swelling. Also, it has caused you to be septic. It is incredible you can walk and talk. Generally, people in your situation would be brought here by ambulance because they had passed out from pain and sepsis. You're going to need emergency surgery. If we don't act fast, you are going to die," he said.

"Okay."

That's really all I had to say. I had an answer. Now I needed a solution. Ask me about Diabetes, and I could tell you everything you wanted to know and how to treat it. But, surgery, kidney stones, and sepsis were all new to me. All I knew was that it had to be done or I wouldn't be able to keep going, and I had things I still wanted to accomplish. There was nothing I could do except agree to the surgery. I couldn't ask for a second opinion. I couldn't sleep on it and see how I felt in the morning.

"The thing is...we only have a general surgeon on premises. It would be preferable if you had a urologist complete the surgery because they are the specialists who do these types of surgeries, but the general surgeon can see you sooner and do the same job," the doctor told me.

The doctor continued to explain how the surgery would work. Even in my morphine haze, I knew I wanted—no, I needed—to be seen by a urologist. I knew from family experience that medical emergencies required the right person for the job to have the best outcome.

"I want a urologist," I replied.

"You'll have to wait until we can call one in to see you," the doctor said.

"Okay, well, am I going to die? Because you just said I needed emergency surgery or I'll die," I asked, my tone even.

"We'll admit you, monitor you very closely, and administer antibiotics and fluids. We will try to keep your pain low enough so you can endure it and get you that urologist," the doctor assured me.

I asked the nurse to hand me my phone, so I could text my parents to tell them what was going on. My mom called me back immediately. She told me she was looking up flights to get to me, but the departures were not early enough. She and my grandma Matilda decided they were going to drive to Phoenix. I told her that wasn't necessary, but she wouldn't hear of it.

"Brandon, this is major surgery. I will be there," she said. I suppose she thought the worst. I knew this surgery was something that needed to be done. Maybe it was the shock of needing serious immediate emergency surgery while facing death. Perhaps I didn't have enough time to process everything, but at the time I did not feel the need to fuss about the seriousness of it all. I just wanted to get back to life as usual.

I'm Still Kickin'

As I waited for the urologist, I became a specimen of interest to much of the hospital staff. Apparently, what I had was rare and the fact that I was alive and talking was some sort of miracle. The next morning, the urologist arrived on site and I was prepped for surgery. They told me that my kidney could burst at any moment and I would die. And, I had less than a 10 percent survival rate if the sepsis escaped the kidney. That seemed extreme, but I knew they were right. *Get me into surgery*, I thought.

I laid on the hospital bed watching the lights above me float past as the orderlies wheeled me to the operating room. Everything looked so white, so sterile, so cold. For the first time since I could remember, I started to feel some kind of emotion creep to the surface...*possibly fear?* On one hand, I just wanted everything to be over. I had secured an internship at law school and didn't want to miss any of my work. I wanted them to blast the kidney stones and shrink the kidney back to its normal size, so I could get back to my life.

On the other hand, I entertained the thought of how I'd feel if I didn't make it out alive. I was very comfortable with how I lived my life thus far. I felt I did everything how I was supposed to – but it wasn't without regret. I had lingering anger and bitterness about my family's betrayal. I had been forced to figure out so much of life on my own; no one did it for me or helped me. I didn't regret that, but I did regret how much time and effort I had spent in pushing down on being mad at the world and feeling bitterness toward people. So much had happened to my family that shaped my attitude toward others. I had spent years keeping people at arm's length. As I awaited my anesthesia, I regretted the ironclad walls I had built around my heart.

If I make it through this, I'm going to do things differently. Walls will fall.

They transported me onto the cold operating table. I counted backwards and fell asleep.

The next thing I remember is waking up extremely tired and desperately wanting to go back to sleep. It was the kind of feeling you get when you fall asleep just moments before your alarm clock goes off. I wanted to hit snooze.

"Brandon! Brandon! Open your eyes! Brandon!" I heard someone yelling. I groaned. Why couldn't I just sleep a little more?

"Brandon!" I heard my name again.

Okay, fine. I thought. My eyes slowly fluttered open in the bright light of the recovery room. I blinked a few times, trying to get rid of the blur as the faces around me started getting clearer. But, my eyes were heavy and needed to be closed again. The doctor shined a bright light into my eyes.

"He's up," someone said.

Someone else handed me a small cup of liquid and told me to drink. It was Diet Coke. I heard someone mumble something about how it would perk me up and irritate my bladder. Why did I want to irritate my bladder?

Gradually things started to make sense. The memory of the excruciating pain came back to the forefront of my mind. I had surgery. I had surgery! That's right!

"Was it successful?" I croaked.

"Yes, everything went well. You were under anesthesia longer than anticipated, which is why we had to make sure you woke up properly."

The doctors explained that they had removed both kidney stones and I was no longer septic. After putting in a stent and draining everything, my kidney was expected to return to normal size. Once the doctors were sure I was lucid, they let my mom and grandma come in to see me. I was so happy to see them. I was happy to be alive. But most of all, I was happy it was over. I wanted to get back to my law school internship before I missed too much work.

Little did I know what this one kidney stone surgery would set in motion.

CHAPTER 2
Highs and Lows

I grasped the sides of the toilet as I projectile vomited once more. Sometimes I couldn't even make it to the toilet in time. Ever since my surgery I got terrible upset stomach aches and the worst nausea possible. A nurse explained the nausea was a common side effect of anesthesia. *Good to know, because vomiting after abdominal surgery is not fun.* The medicine they kept dosing me with through my IV was of no help, unfortunately. But after three days in the hospital I was finally discharged and returned to my apartment and internship. My mom and grandma Matilda went back to California once they were sure I was back on my feet. It had been so good to have them with me and reminded me of the days when I was a kid.

*   *   *

Growing up, my mom and dad always took the best care of me. We were a close-knit family living on a small 10-acre egg ranch between Los Angeles and San Diego. The ranch was magnificent.

From rare goats that looked like sheep mixed with mountain goats to our donkey and cows, it was like a kid's dream. We had plenty of chickens, of course. Every day from sunup to sun down, my dad worked on the ranch to make sure everything looked perfect. The ranch was always pristine. That meant no trash, no weeds, and a perfect lawn. Beyond the aesthetics he meticulously ensured the ranch ran smoothly to produce our eggs. We delivered eggs all over southern California and had an egg store on the ranch where people traveled from all over to buy our fresh eggs. Visitors also enjoyed feeding our goats out front and interacting with our other animals.

The ranch was made up of several barns, each serving their own specific purpose. We had a barn for raising baby chicks, a barn for laying hens, a barn for storing eggs, and, of course, the egg room that housed our packing machine. The machine would suck up a flat of 30 eggs and wash them before continuing on a conveyor belt. Then each egg went through a lighting system to check for cracks or blood. We'd pull the defective eggs off and weigh the acceptable specimens to determine if the egg was extra-large, large, medium, or small. Organized by size and ready to go, the sorted eggs would continue down conveyor belts to be packed into cartons. Then those cartons were boxed, packaged, and delivered to our customers. It was a methodical process.

The ranch was the perfect place for me to grow up. Even from a very young age, I always wanted to help my parents with any task, big or small. Out of nowhere, Mom noticed I became extremely lethargic. In addition to this troubling transformation, I was drinking a lot of water. So much that my mom said I stood by the water dispenser in the kitchen and drank endlessly. I had to pee at twenty-minute intervals throughout the day. My parents called the pediatrician who told them to take me to the best children's hospital in the area, Loma Linda University Medical Center in Loma Linda. That's where I was diagnosed with juvenile diabetes (now called Type 1 Diabetes) and told I'd be insulin dependent for the rest of my life.

Ever the diligent parents, they always kept a close eye on me. It wasn't that they were strict, but rather, they wanted to be sure my diabetes was in check. When I was in 3rd grade, Dr. Smith, my endocrinologist, encouraged me to attend a diabetic camp for a week over the summer. I was so excited. For the first time in my young life, I was away from home and on my own. It was surprising to me how quickly I adapted to being independent. It came naturally to me, even though I was somewhere entirely foreign. Being away from the ranch and from my family gave me the chance to discover who Brandon Mouw was outside of my "ranch bubble."

High in the southern California mountains, the camp reminded me of the mountain towns where I'd deliver eggs with my dad. Tall green pine trees, fresh mountain smell, and dry sandy soil. My family dropped me off in a park area and I boarded a bus that would take me and the other campers to the actual headquarters up in the mountains. I nestled into my seat and quickly learned the people running the camp knew what they were doing. They walked down the aisle handing out snacks, water, and diet soda... typical needs for diabetics. I shouldn't have been surprised but it was reassuring, nonetheless.

As I sat there, I heard the bass and muffled lyrics of different types of music blaring from other campers' headphones. I caught snippets of rap songs about getting high, music I had never heard before. *What was I getting myself into?*

Two hours later, we arrived at the campground. Everything was old-timey and made out of pine wood. I was assigned a cabin with eight other diabetics my age from all over the state. We also had a camp counselor, someone older likely in high school, who would be our leader, so to speak. In the middle of camp, doctors and nurses provided each camper with their insulin injections as well as instructions on how to do it ourselves. There were tons of activities we could sign up for each day like hiking, kayaking, and scavenger hunts. The camp seemed to bring together people from all walks of life. It was unlike anything I've ever experienced before. I was fascinated. It was like I stepped into a different world.

On the second night of camp, I witnessed another diabetic have a low blood sugar episode. All of a sudden, the medical team descended on the cabin and the lights came on. They gave my fellow bunkmate glucagon. It was frightening to see someone unresponsive. *This is what it must be like when my parents would wake me up to drink juice or give me a glucagon shot due to low blood sugar.* I didn't experience emergencies enough to think something was wrong on the rare occasions it happened to me. However, I knew low blood sugars were scary and made me feel like crap afterward.

My bunkmate's blood sugar stabilized as the team assessed him before encouraging us all to go back to sleep. Apparently, the medical team would have people walk around to check on each camper through the night. I was never woken up to test my blood, but we did check our blood sugars before bed and reported them to the counselor.

The first time I went hiking with a group of campers, we got to cross a creek by foot and learn about different parts of nature. We made our own hiking sticks and picked out a special sugar snack to take along for the hike. I even went on a cool hike that took us to an old airplane crash site. You could see where it had hit, slid, and stayed. It sat there, rusted in its resting space. It was like something out of a movie.

Highs and Lows

Every night there was a campfire, glow in the dark games, and night time tag for campers to participate in. There was never a shortage of things to do. Some kids partook and others did their own things. Once I made a few friends, we would go exploring or talk to girls, or try to set traps for snakes. We were just normal kids who happened to have diabetes.

The food was shockingly terrible, and the cafeteria always smelled sweet. At breakfast, lunch, and dinner, I always caught a whiff of that syrupy air. They served scrambled eggs for breakfast. I dared to try them, not really sure what I was eating. They were light yellow, not the rich sunny orange color that I was used to with the fresh eggs from the ranch. I found the camp eggs to be disgusting, but my fellow campers ate them with delight. I later found out when I worked in a summer camp that eggs would be liquefied and placed into bags to be boiled in order to make "scrambled eggs." I guess what we don't know doesn't hurt us. Instead, I opted for peanut butter and jelly sandwiches for just about every meal.

The exposure to life outside the ranch did not overpower my love for back home. I missed my family and the ranch but not to a level of homesickness. Instead, I wrote my parents letters, since we could only use the camp's phone for true emergencies. On the final day of camp, big buses took everyone down the mountain to the drop-off point where all the parents were waiting to pick up their kids. Before we departed, I exchanged addresses and phone numbers with my new friends so we could keep in touch.

As I jumped off the bus, I found my mom, dad, and siblings eagerly awaiting my arrival with big smiles on their faces.

This was my first time away from home, so they were relieved to see I was in one piece.

"How was it, Brandon?" my mom asked me.

"It was awesome! We fished and I got to watch a talent show!" I exclaimed happily. I learned so much about Diabetes management and I left with a newfound sense of confidence about controlling my illness. Not to mention I had a ton of fun.

I still have a photo of me hugging my siblings as if we hadn't seen each other in years! That week was one I will never forget.

*   *   *

From diabetic camp on, I took excellent care of my health because I learned how to manage my disease on my own. I was rarely sick. The only time I missed school was for a doctor's appointment or the time I had chickenpox. Otherwise, I was very healthy. Feeling ill and even needing surgery were foreign to me. Yet here I was, healing from my kidney surgery, and feeling as if something was off. It was frustrating.

Just days after I was discharged from the hospital, I noticed the left side of my back was black, blue and very swollen. *Wasn't all the surgery internal?* I thought. Maybe the swelling caused some discoloration. It did not look pretty. At least I was not in the hospital though, and could finish my internship.

Exactly one week later, I returned to the doctor for my follow-up appointment. My surgeon assured me everything was fine, and the bruising was completely normal. I took his word for it. But I quickly learned that things were not completely normal.

Shortly after the follow-up appointment, I started feeling unwell, just not my normal self. All my life I had high and low blood sugar episodes, so I was accustomed to the ebbs and flows of my health. When a low blood sugar hit, my energy would be zapped. I would feel my lips tingle. My vision would be off. I would lose track of time and feel extremely lethargic. My heart would beat fast as my body tried to process blood and get carbohydrates and sugars out of it. My chest would feel empty and I wouldn't even notice my lungs filling up because my heart was beating so fast. Plus, I'd be confused. It would be as if my brain just wasn't catching on. I'd have to find sugar, juice, candy, or food. Growing up, my mom and dad would usually get me to eat something to bring my sugar up. A normal blood sugar is around 100. A low blood sugar is below 70, and a high blood sugar is above 160.

A high blood sugar brought on a whole new bout of symptoms. My vision wouldn't be good, and I'd feel very hot, sweaty, and uncomfortable. My mouth would dry up, and I'd get very short and crabby with people. I knew I needed to bring down the blood sugar with insulin. I would test my blood to confirm my suspicion. Like a roller coaster, there were ups and downs and proper ways to treat a high or low blood sugar. It was always a delicate balance between the two diabetic outcomes.

I started having more lows. Imagine you're going, going, going and then suddenly you just crash. Speech starts to slur as if you are drunk. The brain shuts down other non-essential functions to preserve energy for the heart and lungs. It's scary and confusing and feels terrible. For me, it usually took my body at least six to eight hours to rest and recover mentally and physically from the crash.

I had experienced this sensation many times before, but it started to happen more frequently. I didn't have the mental and physical energy I did before the kidney stones. I'd wake up in the middle of the night with low blood sugar (about 50) and knock things over in my apartment as I scrambled in the dark to find one of my orange Gatorades, my trusty low blood sugar treatment.

One day during my law internship, I started to feel off. My vision started to blur and everything felt strange, like I was in an altered reality. I reached under my desk into my bag in search of my Gatorade. But there wasn't any left. *What the hell?* I thought. I always brought plenty to work with me. It hadn't occurred to me that I blew through my stash. I reached into the side pocket in search of my backup candy, Mentos, but I was met with an empty wrapper. It was the first time, in my entire life, where I was out of all my low blood sugar supplies. I tend to be organized and on top of it, so I was shocked that I didn't even realize when I had run out of my emergency supply. I knew something was seriously wrong. I found something to snack on in the office and called my doctor to explain what happened. They got me in for their very next appointment – two months later.

The low blood sugar episodes happened unpredictably and very quickly, without warning. I would eat lunch and immediately have low blood sugar, not because I gave myself too much insulin too soon, but for no reason at all. Normally a person wouldn't have low blood sugar for a few hours after eating because the body has fuel. But, I'd eat my meal, not take insulin, and still would crash immediately. I did my best to control the low blood sugars as I finished the weeks left of my internship.

When I finally had my appointment with my endocrinologist, I explained exactly what was happening. She lowered my insulin dose, more than I had done myself, thinking that had contributed to the low blood sugars, but it didn't make a difference.

"Brandon, eat a graham cracker before bed," my endocrinologist told me. That was the medical advice I received. Eat a graham cracker. *That certainly would solve all my problems*, I thought to myself sarcastically. It did not surprise me that I found myself returning to the doctor's office two weeks later, still having the same symptoms. They lowered my insulin again, changed brands, and told me to eat more often. I did what they told me to do, but even on my good days, I wasn't feeling quite right.

I went to my primary care doctor again, because the endocrinologist thought it had to be something else contributing to the low blood sugars, and I once again explained all the symptoms I had been having. I asked my doctor to run some lab work. Everything came back normal. I returned two weeks later, demanding answers. I had no energy to do anything at all. Low blood sugars were hitting me hard and taking a toll on me. I felt like weights were literally holding me down when I tried to move. My eyes felt heavy, my body felt like it was being attacked.

"Oh, your blood pressure is really high, Brandon," my primary care doctor said. "Let's up your blood pressure medicine. That should do the trick."

We did. I started at 10mg, then 20mg, and eventually 40mg. My symptoms remained and I got worse. The doctors were not catching on to what I was saying. They couldn't quantify it. Red lights and alarms should have been going off the whole time but none of the health professionals were listening.

It was a tell-tale sign of what was to come. Little did I know this was just the beginning of what I'd consider to be the biggest and hardest struggle of my entire life.

CHAPTER 3

I Am Not Okay

It got to the point where I knew I had to become my own advocate. I made the decision to speak up for myself because no one else was going to. If anything, after my first kidney issue, I learned that if I didn't ask for something then it was easy for people in the medical field to forget about important things. I knew I needed to be heard and understood from now on. No more dilly-dallying around. The doctors kept reassuring me that I was fine. My primary care doctor, a general practitioner, told me, "This is just the best you are going to live. It's not bad." They kept tweaking my medications and requesting follow-up appointments, but I had had enough.

"I'm not leaving this office without an order for an ultrasound, CT scan, X-ray, or MRI of my kidneys, organs, or anything else that can be wrong," I said with finite determination. The labs were not enough. This wasn't worth beating around the bush anymore. I needed to find out what was wrong and wouldn't accept no as an answer.

"Your kidney function looks great in your labs," my doctor said.

"I had kidney surgery. Nothing we're doing is working or giving us answers. I continually get worse. I need something done immediately," I said sternly.

Since my first surgery, my nephrologist (kidney doctor) said my kidney function was fine. My labs said my kidney function was slightly elevated, but that was more than likely from being a diabetic for more than 25 years, so it was just fine. My doctors said my kidneys were in great shape, all things considered.

She reluctantly agreed to order an ultrasound. She was probably hoping to prove me wrong and shut me up. Who was I to demand such a thing? The appointment was set for a Thursday in December 2015.

The day after the ultrasound, my nephrologist called me. "You need to come into the office today, Brandon."

"I don't have an appointment until after the New Year," I replied.

"It doesn't matter. You're in kidney failure. You need emergency surgery." he said. *Here we go again.*

My nephrologist admitted me to the hospital and made a few calls to a urologist he trusted who could complete the surgery. I would have to be in the hospital for at least a week. My exams were looming and I really didn't like having to drop everything for an emergency surgery. My doctor told me to go grab a few things from home, make sure to bring my books to study, and go to the hospital right away. My surgeon would be waiting for me the moment I stepped through the door.

I had no choice. If I postponed, I would only get worse and maybe die. I went home and collected a few things before heading to the hospital. I didn't have time to process what was happening. I wasn't scared. I just knew I had to get it done.

As I walked through the now familiar doors, the sterile scent of disinfectant hit my nose. The staff already had a bed ready for me. I let my mom know what was going on and told her she did not need to drive to Arizona like last time. She was worried, but told me I would be okay. To my surprise, the nurses took me up right away, anticipating my arrival. I thought, *this must be really serious.* They helped me prep for surgery. I changed into a hospital gown and put my belongings in a bag for safekeeping. I signed a few forms and the urologist arrived to explain what was going to happen.

"Your kidney is blocked again, most likely from another stone or even one from the previous surgery," he said. "We're going to do exactly what you had done before and it shouldn't take long." Before I knew it, I was carted off to the operating room. It felt like déjà vu, or Groundhog Day.

"We're going to put you under now," was the last thing I remember hearing before waking up groggily and blinking my eyes several times to help them focus.

It took me a few minutes to recall where I was and what I was doing there in the first place. Then it hit me. *Kidney failure. Emergency surgery. Hospital.*

"Was it successful?" I asked the navy scrubs floating around the room. The nurses were clearly dodging me and my question.

"No," someone finally answered.

"What do you mean, NO?" I asked, opening my eyes wider and looking around.

"The surgeon will be in shortly to talk to you," someone to my left replied. I closed my eyes, wondering if the surgery was unsuccessful, what would be next? *Was I truly in jeopardy of death?* Would I be able to take my law school examinations on time? Should my mom have come to the hospital this time? I had told her not to worry.

"Hello, Brandon." I heard a voice coming from my doorway. It was my surgeon, the one recommended by my nephrologist.

"You have something, I'm assuming some sort of scar tissue, between your kidney and your ureter, which is the duct that allows urine to pass from the kidneys to the bladder," he explained. "The scar tissue was too hard for our strongest surgical tools to remove. We couldn't even obtain a sample for testing. Your urine has caused your kidney to enlarge to the size of an inflated balloon. We must drain your kidney."

I processed this information for a moment before asking the million-dollar question. "Why couldn't you drain my kidney during this surgery?"

"I'm sorry," he explained. "We didn't have a release form to insert a nephrectomy tube and drain your kidney from your back. After being under anesthesia, the protocol is that patients can no longer make legal decisions for 12 hours. We needed your next of kin to approve the procedure."

Well that's stupid and negligent and a terrible way to handle such a serious situation, I angrily thought. I understood laws were laws, but due to this one, I was denied a life-saving medical procedure. With no other option on hand, I had to contact my mom and have her talk to the doctor and legal department over the phone, granting the medical team permission to insert the tube so my kidney could drain. This also meant I'd have to go in for a second surgery that night.

While my mom had several back and forth calls with the powers that be, the nurses checked on me often to make sure I wasn't poisoned to death by my balloon of a kidney that was on the verge of bursting at any time. When the release for the nephrectomy tube surgery was confirmed, I returned to the operating room once more. This time they put me under local anesthesia, a twilight sleep, instead of knocking me out completely.

"Okay," I vaguely heard the surgeon say. When I woke up, I felt the tube projecting from my back. It was attached to a bag on my side, similar to a catheter bag. A nurse held up the bag, examining its contents. It was full of blood.

"Is that normal?" I asked her.

She smiled at me sympathetically. "Everything looks okay for now. Your kidney is draining."

I was ready to get out of there. I had to take my finals, get ready and pack because there was somewhere important I had to be that January 7th. During my first year of law school, I had applied for this internship. Washington, D.C. was at the top of my list. After applications and interviews, I was offered a second internship, this time with a member in the House of Representatives in their legal department. I also applied for an internal law program in D.C. through my law school. I got the green light on both opportunities. For the first time in my life, I'd have the chance to experience the East Coast! It was a life experience I did not want to miss. How could such good things and bad things be happening at the same time?

But, my kidney had other plans for me. I had to get *yet another* surgery. The surgeon wanted to go through the hole in my back, through the kidney, and break up the scar tissue with wires to clear the pathway through my ureter. Somehow that tissue was stronger than any wire, tool, or laser they had and the surgery was a total failure. The scar tissue remained, and the surgeon had to go back to the drawing board.

Each surgery felt more painful than the last. I was getting frustrated. I continued to feel like crap as the doctors tried to come up with a plan to fix me. Law school exams came and went. Thankfully the doctors sent my law school registrar a medical note explaining my extreme circumstances. The note would allow me to take my exams between surgeries. Not ideal, but I had no other options.

My life began to look something like this: I'd go to the hospital for my procedure and spend a few nights in recovery before returning home. After that, I'd return for my follow-up as the doctors tried to figure out what was next. Most students had finished for the semester, which was a blessing in disguise. When I went in to take my exams, knowing I probably wouldn't do well, I sat in a room all alone. I had a tube protruding from my back, which was attached to a bag filled with blood and urine. It was the perfect conversation starter, but there was no one around to talk to. It wasn't attractive and I'm sure if people saw me they thought I was crazy, but I had goals to achieve. I had no time for this kidney ordeal to hold me back.

After finals, the doctors set me up for another surgery. This time they wanted to put in a larger tube to help my kidney drain better, faster, and possibly serve as a long-term solution. I literally had a PVC pipe sticking out of my back. It was angled toward my left side and attached to what looked like a garden hose affixed to a large bag. The goal was to keep this larger tube in place for three months before it could be removed.

I Am Not Okay

"I'm leaving on January 7th for an internship and classes in Washington, D.C.," I said. "Do what you have to do to make that happen, but I'm not missing my flight. I have a chance of a lifetime, and I am not going to let your inability to remove scar tissue from my kidney stop me. Expecting me to have this tube that requires a nurse to flush and clean it out while being on the other side of the country is also out of the question."

When I updated my family, my mom protested at my determination. Was I demanding a lot? Yes. Asking for the impossible to be done? Absolutely not. I knew this was serious, but also solvable. I had put so much effort into everything I had done to accomplish my goals. I had finally found something, in law school, that I loved and gave me purpose again. I was determined to overcome this latest health challenge. I was healthy, never needed medical intervention before, and it had been a long time since I woke up each morning, excited for the day to come.

*   *   *

The last time I felt this excitement was when I was a kid growing up on the egg ranch. I remember every afternoon when I came home from school, I tossed my backpack in my room and ran out to the ranch to see what else needed to be done. There was never a shortage of work, which was great. Sometimes I'd hose down the egg store parking lot, make sure the chicken building lights were timed correctly, or repair something that had broken. My heart was full. I relished every single minute of it. No matter what I did, I felt pride and accomplishment.

As I grew older, I earned more responsibility. I cared for the chickens and animals, worked with customers in the egg store, helped with egg packing, and went on deliveries with my dad. I remember one winter, when I was about five years old, my dad and

I headed to the mountains for a delivery and the egg van got stuck in the snow.

"I'll get the snow chains," my dad said as he hopped out of the driver's seat. I sat quietly in the passenger's seat, waiting for direction. My dad fumbled with the chains for a moment before hopping back up on the driver's side and opening the door.

"Brandon, will you move over and press the gas and then the brake so I can get the chain secured?" my dad asked.

"Yes!" I said enthusiastically. I would do anything to help out my dad. I climbed out of my seat and huddled on the driver's side floor. Hands at the ready, I waited for my dad's instructions.

"Pull the gear to drive and gently push the gas," my dad said. "Now stop!" he shouted over the engine noise. Diligently, I obeyed. "Got it!"

I don't know many parents who would instruct their five-year-old kid to put a van in gear and operate the pedals, but we got it done and finished the deliveries in the mountains. It meant a lot to me that my dad trusted me to complete such an adult task. He didn't think twice.

He knew I could do it. My dad is the kindest and hardest working person I have ever known. Before he began suffering from depression, he always had a special spark for life. He made sure our lives were polar opposite from his upbringing. Despite getting up early to start up the egg machine, run a business, and staying up late to wrap things up on the ranch, my dad always would set time aside to play with us. He taught us how to ride a bike and how to golf, which was his passion. As the egg farm became more successful, my parents took us on bigger and longer vacations. When I showed an interest in birds, my parents got an aviary built on the ranch. They made sure the entire family had fun and wanted for nothing.

Each morning my mom got us ready for school. We ate breakfast (nothing beats fresh eggs in the morning), got dressed, and piled into the car. School was about a 30-minute drive from the ranch, so we'd have to get up early and be ready so as not to be late. I didn't care much for school. Grades didn't mean anything to me.

If we go to school to learn things that prepare us for our careers as adults, I was in the wrong place. When I was younger, all I wanted to do was eventually take over the family egg business. Besides some basic math and writing, school did next to nothing to prepare me for that career. I had everything I needed back at home. My dad was the best role model, and each day I learned something new about running a business. The ranch was my school and I knew I'd make a great egg rancher and businessman...all of that would soon change.

*   *   *

That's why law school was now so important to me. I was, somehow, good at it. I was excited to wake up each morning. I saw purpose in a way I hadn't since those years growing up on the egg ranch. And, I was thriving. This stupid kidney was not going to get in the way.

Resolute with my decision to go to D.C., I stuck with my timeline. At every chance I got, I told each nurse and doctor I had to be out there on January 7th so they better have a solution to the problem. I tried to be firm, but respectful and clear about my intentions. Truthfully, I just wanted to advocate for myself and make sure everyone understood my goal. My medical team worked hard to come up with a solution that would allow me to fly out to D.C. on time.

To help me meet my deadline, the doctors tried a different technique. Using a two-prong approach with stronger tools, they went through my back and up through my urethra with lasers and wires and metal devices to break up the scar tissue. It failed. And it was painful when I woke up. I never complained. I just took each procedure with stride, knowing it was something that had to be done no matter the pain or cost. However, I was getting tired of being prepped and having different tools and wires and tubes dug into me. It felt like I had taken up residence in the hospital at that point. Having my blood drawn daily every day was one thing I couldn't get over. Something about the cold needles being stuck in my veins took me right back to that scared three-year-old boy being pinned down on that hospital table all those years ago. It's funny how memories stick around.

The doctors treated my case as the ultimate medical mystery challenge while I started packing up for my internship. My mom took me shopping while I had a large bag tied to my waist. The bag was collecting urine and blood from the tubing in my back, helping drain the kidney. Not the best of circumstances, but I didn't care. My mom did everything to help me get the supplies I'd need for my upcoming semester. When my professors notified me that I had passed my law finals, I knew my hard work had paid off. It felt so good as I completed my preliminary checklist for D.C., making sure that things like security clearances, background checks, and various applications were all in order.

When I returned for my next appointment, my trusty surgeon had a new idea he wanted to try, since by now they had exhausted most traditional surgical options. He thought it best to leave the second large nephrostomy tube in my back for six months to see what my kidney did on its own. We discussed that a late 20-something year old should not be in this situation and the expectation of keeping the tube in my back for longer than absolutely necessary was not appropriate.

"Okay Brandon, we're going to go in laparoscopically and remove the scar tissue from the kidney and ureter. We'll reattach everything and sew you up. You will be able to go to D.C. by February," they told me.

I laughed. "Sounds like a plan, but all that has to be done ASAP as I'm leaving January 7th."

"That's impossible. The recovery time is months, and we need to book specialized equipment for this procedure."

"I'm leaving, so what do I need to do to make this happen?" I asked harshly.

Next thing I knew, somehow, even though the scheduler said it was an impossible task, they reserved the da Vinci laparoscopy machine, for the day before Christmas.

I walked into the hospital once more. They prepped me for surgery, a routine I had memorized by now. I changed into my hospital gown and laid down on the transport bed. As they wheeled me down the hall to the operating room I felt at peace. This had to work. I was on a mission.

The surgeons removed one-quarter of my kidney. They meticulously cleared the scar tissue, cut off the part of the ureter bound with scar tissue, and reattached it all. Knowing I'd be flying across the country "no matter what," my incisions were closed with dissolvable stitches and glue instead of the traditional method using staples. Now I wouldn't have to return until the stent had to be removed from my bladder. It would be a simple procedure I could schedule over a weekend later down the line.

I'm Still Kickin'

Merry Christmas to me. Everyone worked with me to get it done. I was thankful. Being a solid patient advocate was the only way this would work and I just might have made it happen... maybe.

CHAPTER 4

The Capitol

After another successful surgery, I sat in a tiny hospital room recovering, waiting for the swelling to go down, the kidney creatinine to drop, and the drain to clear of bloody fluids. Every day I asked if I could please be released. I couldn't wait to escape the bright white walls and pastel window curtains. I was alive and ready for my next adventure.

It was late in the afternoon on January 5th when I was given the green light to leave the hospital. I'd have to return on Valentine's Day, about six weeks out, to have my stent removed. *I could do that.* Luckily, my mom had come over from California and helped me pack the remainder of my things for D.C.. I couldn't lift anything. I had just undergone seven surgeries in a very short amount of time. She even had to carry my suitcases to the car as we left for the airport at 3:00 a.m.

I had a hard time adjusting to feeling so helpless. When I tried to lift even the lightest of items, I couldn't. My kidney and ureter were held together with stitches. My back was sore from all the plumbing I had in it, and I had cuts all over my side and torso that were held together with only dissolvable stitches and glue. I could only imagine what everyone thought about me trying to make all this happen. My mom was phenomenal, and I couldn't have made it to the airport without her. She was so patient and encouraging. I gave up lifting things because I didn't want to hurt myself in any way and cause further delay.

"Mom, I'm going to ask for a wheelchair," I told her as we pulled up to departures. An airport employee arrived by my side and helped me with the luggage as well.

"Have a safe flight," my mom said before gently hugging me goodbye. She thought I was crazy to travel across the country after everything, but she supported me nonetheless. I would not have recovered or made it to the airport without her.

"Thank you for everything, Mom." I meant it.

Mom couldn't fly with me to D.C. and get me set up in my new apartment in a completely new place. With this in mind, I looked up personal assistants on line and found someone I could hire for the day. I sent them a list of grocery items to pick up and bring to the room I would be renting.

"Attention passengers, we will now begin boarding," resonated over the airport intercom.

Given my wheelchair, I received priority boarding. Not a bad perk for someone who had just endured so many surgeries. Once settled in my seat, I looked out the window, excited for what was next. I didn't have any expectations. I knew better than to expect anything, because the unexpected can slap you in the face. It was a painful flight with one layover. Sitting so upright pulled on my wounds and I could feel every bump deep in my body. As I tried to get comfortable, I thought about how this would be my first time to the East Coast. The farthest east I had made it before was a fateful trip to Michigan that triggered a sequence of events that altered the course of my life forever.

*   *   *

I was 15 years old, the ranch was doing really well, and we were all very happy as a family. If Dad wasn't spending time with us or planning our next family vacation, we could find him seeking new investment opportunities or running the egg ranch by phone.

As a kid, you're pretty blind to adult business affairs. While I knew the labor aspects of running an egg ranch, I wasn't privy to the business decisions made behind closed doors. Little did I know, Dad wanted to help out his brothers and his parents in a very big way. Since our egg ranch was doing so well at that time, he wanted to invest and help both his siblings launch their own businesses.

My uncle Walter had made a few bad business decisions with the dairy his wife and her family had owned. Wanting to continue working in the dairy industry, he moved to Washington because he found that it was less expensive to start over there. My other uncle, Luke, who was recently married, also worked for his in-law's dairy. He learned that if he could come up with about $100,000, he could get his own dairy in Washington, too.

Uncle Walter went into business with my grandparents to get his dairy going with the agreement that my grandparents receive a $10,000 a month guaranteed income from it. Then, when my uncle and grandparents asked Dad to loan them money to get by, he did so without hesitation. Dad was never greedy or selfish. He just wanted the best for everyone and saw an opportunity to help his family. As if on cue, Uncle Luke also asked Dad for financial help. He needed an investment loan totaling $100,000 to get his dairy off the ground in Washington. Dad wrote a check and gave it to him, supposedly creating a partnership. The deal was that Dad owned half the dairy. While uncle Luke paid back the $100,000 five years later, Dad did not receive any profits from the dairy or interest on the loan. Still, Dad kept his brother and parents afloat, on top of managing our own ranch back in California.

When my grandparents needed to prove they had $10,000 a month in income for three years to take out a loan for a chicken ranch in Iowa, they turned to my ever-so-generous dad. Their dairy did not produce enough profit to support my uncle's family and my grandparents' guaranteed income. Dad knew it. He put money in their bank account, so they could say they had the monthly $10,000 to open their new business. My grandparents even stole $500,000 in cash from my dad under the guise of a cow purchase for their dairy. Instead of cows, they bought a motorhome and housing lots on a golf course in Washington. Dad didn't complain because he just wanted to see everyone succeed. He also wanted to keep the peace in the family, because there was never peace when he was growing up.

If you do the math, you can see Dad loaned out incredibly large sums of money to the family. Most of those loans were never paid back. It was the ultimate betrayal, both for Dad and for my immediate family. I think he chalked it up as a loss without realizing his generosity may have been the biggest mistake he ever made. Nothing could have prepared us for the huge pitfalls we would face because of Dad's big heart. Nothing.

The beginning of the end of the egg ranch happened when my family and I flew to Michigan, to visit my aunt on my mom's side, with my maternal grandparents and two cousins in tow. We went golfing, jet skiing, fishing, boating, wakeboarding, tubing, and played cards every night. Three days into our trip, however, I was fishing at the lake with my cousins when I realized Dad had yet to join us. He never missed a jet ski excursion or a fishing expedition.

"Mom, where's Dad?" I asked her, perplexed by his absence.

"He's on the phone. Said he had to take a call," she replied.

It wasn't unusual for him to step aside and take a business call about the ranch. After all, even if we were on vacation, the ranch still ran and our employees packed and delivered eggs for our customers. My cousins and I continued fishing until it was time to return to my aunt and uncle's place.

Mom brought my brother, sister, and I back to the hotel room. As we opened the door, we found Dad standing there, packed, and ready to leave.

"Where are you going?" I asked him.

"I'm sorry, I have to head back to the ranch," he said. "I just got a call that our largest account dropped us. I need to head back to figure out what is going on."

Dad delivered the news with calm precision, not wanting to upset us or "ruin" our vacation. But I could tell it was more serious than he was letting on. We just bought the pullets (young chickens about to start laying quality eggs) to keep our supply consistent and leased a ranch that was four times the size of our original property.

What did this mean?

Dad said goodbye to us and walked out to the car. He told us to continue having fun and not to worry about anything. But, I could tell my parents seemed worried. It would be hard to have fun knowing something serious was happening back home. It was even harder knowing I was apart from Dad and not able to step in to help. The remainder of our trip passed by in a blur.

Our family had a longstanding relationship with the family behind the account that dropped us—of more than 15 years. Dad started supplying their eggs when they had only one store. Now they had over 20 grocery stores and we'd deliver a truckload of eggs every other day to each store. We were invited to their family birthdays and parties. When we would go snowboarding, we'd take their son, who was my age. Dad shared his favorite pastime with the company's owner, teaching him to golf like the pros. We delivered eggs in snow and on holidays, even at Christmas. We had provided them with the most exceptional service for a decade and a half. We treated them like family and vice versa, at least until that day in Michigan when they called my dad and said, "Don't bring us any more eggs."

Our accounts had 90 days to pay the "egg invoice" after delivery. Instead of saying "in 90 days we're switching suppliers," which would provide us a three-month cushion to find new clients, this company pulled the rug out from under our feet—overnight and with no warning. They gave us no real reason for this instantaneous change. It was the worst possible timing. We had just bought pullets and leased a larger ranch. We had a feed truck that came by every other day with over $100,000 worth of prepaid feed for the chickens. A chicken lays about an egg a day, and we had a lot of chickens. We were processing tons of eggs and did not have enough clients to purchase the supply. The eggs can only stay in a cooler for so long. Our ranch only had so much storage. We needed to find a home for the surplus—and fast. Twenty grocery store deliveries worth of surplus.

First, Dad tried to find new customers who would be willing to buy the eggs. Unfortunately for us, there weren't any egg shortages happening in the country. There were no new big clients and no clusters of smaller stores in the market for eggs because they already had suppliers. We weren't used to it, but we were forced to go to the Los Angeles markets and sell eggs wholesale at a fraction of the market price. We still had our smaller clients and our egg store, but it failed to put even the slightest dent in our growing egg collection. It didn't take long for the panic set in. You really see how much money gets blown in a day when you don't see the return on investment. The money we spent to keep the ranch running quickly exceeded our profits and broke into our savings.

After that large account dropped us, I went from ranch to ranch, making sure everything was good until one day Dad told me not to go to the other ranch anymore. He had sold all of the pullets for pennies on the dollar for what he paid for them. Then, he broke the lease on the larger ranch. He still had to pay the lease in full, plus additional fees. In his mind, it was the only thing he could do to stop the hemorrhaging of cash. I knew things were bad, but I just did what he asked of me. I knew better than to weigh in on some of Dad's decisions. I trusted him and my mom to work things out and get us back on the right path. My parents had enough cash on hand to pay off our houses, cars, education, and the broken lease for the large egg ranch while maintaining our smaller local accounts. If we reduced our staff, we could have kept our heads above water, but we were still struggling. Lost, with the glimpse of failure on the horizon, we didn't know what to do next. Dad called his parents, long-time egg ranchers, for advice. He had spent years helping them financially, loaning and even giving away money without a second thought. Instead of business advice or even a little financial assistance, he was told off. The same people he lent money to so they could get through their own financial difficulties were the same people who basically said, "Screw you, figure it out."

He reached out to other family members, the people to whom he lent millions of dollars so they could get their respective dairies and businesses off the ground and continue to run when they were short each month. They, too, said they couldn't help. Their many investments my dad had funded went south, or so they said. Nothing was in writing, of course. Nothing except Dad's crisp and clear signature on loan documents for his parents and brothers as cosigners. It was an impossible situation. It was heartbreaking.

I didn't know it at the time, but there was another powerful force playing in the downfall of our finances. The very family members who refused my dad when he needed their help, back when this all began, returned. They came out of the woodwork to request money for all sorts of things under the cloak of "investments." Dad, mentally and physically sick and tired of being bothered by endless phone calls, was signing blank checks and mailing them off to my aunt, my uncle, and my grandparents. We had no idea this was happening until it was too late. He must have thought he was investing money in one of the dairies and other business ventures, like he had been trying to do, but it wasn't until five years later we'd learn that was not the case.

Dad, blinded by optimism, tried to invest in businesses he hoped would boost his income. He invested in a tractor weed abating company. He invested in gas stations. He invested in purchasing milking and beef cows. Nothing worked out. He threw money at whatever he thought could provide a return and came up short each time. It was like tossing spaghetti noodles at the wall, hoping they'd stick, only to watch each one slowly slide down and crumple in a heap on the floor. Nothing worked out.

Desperate to keep food on the table, my parents applied for loans. The problem was our financial history showed we were making a large sum of money and then portrayed an abrupt loss, followed by crippling debt. Before we had to start to sell things off, we owned several properties, animal and farm equity, a portion of a bank, gas stations, two lube stations, investments in two dairies, lots of stock, two egg ranches, and three houses. With each passing day, the assets were sold, and we got dangerously close to having nothing.

I know what it is like to not worry about money and be able to afford to live without want. I know what it is like to be poverty stricken and worry about where my next meal is going to come from. Going from having everything I could want to not even being able to afford to get gas to deliver eggs or buy groceries for the family was a drastic change, especially when it happened practically overnight. But the loss of provisions and material things would not wreak havoc the most on our family. Instead, a silent culprit in the form of Dad's depression contributed to our family's demise and fed my growing resentment.

I worked harder, combing the region to secure new accounts. I didn't want to go to college because I planned on taking over the egg ranch when I graduated high school. I had no idea that dream would become a reality so quickly, and under such dire conditions, but I still loved the work. I wanted to see the ranch succeed and for us, as a family, to overcome this tremendous hurdle—which seemed possible at the time. I suppose I had blinders on and just kept moving forward. If I didn't do it, no one else would.

*   *   *

Maybe this is where my cutthroat determination comes from, I thought as the wintry Chicago skyline came into view. I had a brief layover before continuing on to our nation's Capitol. Despite being physically helpless and in moderate pain, I was going to do whatever it took to get there—come hell or high water.

When the plane landed, I sadly requested another wheelchair realizing how hurt I truly was from just having a major surgery and traveling, and so was carted off to the baggage area. The personal assistant I had hired awaited me, to help me with my bags and drive me to my new apartment, just steps from the Capitol. I didn't know what I would do without help to move my bags, carry groceries, or get around. I found that hiring an assistant for the day would solve all those issues once I arrived in D.C.

After some tricky and slow maneuvering up three flights of narrow row house stairs, I arrived at my home away from home. The assistant carried my luggage up the stairs, unpacked my things, put the groceries away, and even made my bed for me. There was no way I could have made it on my own that first night. After getting everything settled, I paid the assistant, then went to bed. I was in disbelief. I really had made it.

I was in Washington, D.C.! I considered this a huge victory for me in terms of my health and achieving my goals.

CHAPTER 5
Code Blue

For a guy who grew up on a small chicken ranch in California, Washington, D.C. was magnificent. As a law student interning in the heart of all things judicial, I made friends with the people I worked with, as well as others while attending events in the city. It really is an easy place to make friends, which is drastically different than on the West Coast. D.C. culture is inviting, filled with networking opportunities, and making a new friend is as easy as saying hello to the table you're sitting next to at dinner. In southern California, the culture is more laid back, they don't branch out from their normal social circles as willingly, and people mind their own business. In addition, things in California were very spread out. In D.C., you could walk to everything. Hanging out was so simple. We could walk or take the Metro anywhere. The difference is striking. (Even more so when you attended different small Christian schools with a class size of about 18.)

I'm Still Kickin'

Every Friday, my friends and I went to happy hour, dinner, karaoke, saw a concert, or explored somewhere new. For the first time I felt like a normal person, socially. I had a core group of friends I could rely on, including one friend who knew the signs of low blood sugar and would warn me to eat or drink something if he thought I was acting funny. He had a good friend who was a diabetic, so he could recognize if I was low and tell me to eat a Snickers bar. It was nice to know I wasn't alone and that someone else had an idea of what was going on. He did everything on his own, without my asking. He knew what I needed and stepped up to the challenge.

Still, my low blood sugar episodes kept happening. One minute I would be fine and the next minute they would drop without warning. A whole day at my internship could go by and all of a sudden people would ask me, "Hey Brandon, are you going home?" I wouldn't even realize it was evening, nor could I tell you what I had done during the day. I had no clue why or what was going on with my blood sugars.

Searching for a justification, I continued to blame it on my very active and demanding lifestyle. I tried to eat and keep a closer eye on my blood sugar, but it didn't help. I had a continuous glucose monitor (CGM) which read my blood every few minutes and sent the results to a monitor. By the time my monitor would alert me to a low blood sugar, I'd be too far gone mentally to realize it because my blood sugar would drop so suddenly.

Somehow, I didn't let this interfere with my work or social life. I pushed through and told myself that it was all part of the experience. *Nothing prevented me from moving forward before. I had goals to accomplish, so why dwell on it,* I would tell myself. My supervisor continued to assign tasks, and I was able to complete things on time. I had lots of moments where I didn't remember exactly what I did, but I suppose I did it sufficiently because I received no redirects or complaints. I sat in on hearings and took notes. I ran messages back and forth to legislative members. My low blood sugars weren't stopping me. The only people who knew something was up were in my close circle of friends—and even they were only aware of a small portion of what was going on. In fact, I didn't know how bad things truly were. My friends worried to the extent I'd let them. I would have food, juice, or candy with me, and they would remind me to eat it if I started acting goofy or got pale and sweaty.

At the conclusion of that amazing internship and classes, I flew back to Arizona to visit my doctors for a check-up. In a short time, I'd be spending the next three months in D.C. for a prestigious Department of State summer legal internship. *How did I even get accepted?* But first, I had to see my doctor.

"Are you eating the graham cracker before bed?" my endocrinologist asked me.

It felt patronizing. I ate frequently and always had protein and complex carbohydrates before bed to keep my blood sugar from going low. I knew how to take care of myself; I'd been doing it for nearly 30 years at that point. The graham cracker was not going to help. *It wasn't some magic item that solved low blood sugar issues.* I had been diagnosed at age three and never had I ever been hospitalized for my type 1 diabetes. It was just that the low blood sugars continued to hit without warning. Despite this report, my doctors gave me the "all clear." I was told to keep doing what I was doing, continue to eat often, and just live my life. My kidney function was normal, and the low blood sugars remained a diabetic mystery. I was told to maintain as normal a life as possible and be extra purposeful about eating more often. Their nonchalance influenced my own attitude. Maybe it wasn't something to worry about. The doctors blamed it on stress, law school, and my "new environment." They promised that my body would get over it in due time and provided no real or direct answers.

I was always someone who went out of my way to solve a problem and create solutions no matter what effort it took. With no clarity as to what I could do to help myself, I was reminded of having this feeling before: this sense of helplessness when my dad stopped being able to get out of bed. My mom and I tried to seek answers from every doctor, guru, psychologist, and religious clergy to determine what was wrong with him. None of which offered any help or clarity. Few things are as maddening as watching someone fall apart with no remedy in sight. It is something you can never really erase from your mind.

*　　*　　*

At first, I noticed my dad's absence in the evening, when we'd usually be outdoors participating in activities on the ranch. But then he disappeared from work at the egg ranch. And then he disappeared from just about every aspect of life. He was there physically, but he just couldn't get out of bed. He laid there for hours on end with the shades drawn. The phone rang constantly as our workers and customers called about ranch business. Dad ignored them.

When they couldn't reach my dad, they tried to reach me. I'd go to him to relay the message or ask the question on hand, but he was sleeping or silent in his room, which he kept dark all hours of the day. Not wanting the business to stall, I started taking the calls myself and directing everyone as best as I could. I was barely 16, thrown into the full-time duties of running the family's egg ranch.

I wasn't my dad, but he had taught me a lot of chicken business fundamentals growing up. I knew how to produce eggs. I knew how to gain new accounts. I knew how to make deliveries. I knew how to collect money. I knew how to track invoices, and I knew everyone who worked for us, personally.

Dad never asked for a thing in his entire life. He did everything on his own and worked his butt off to provide for everyone he loved. He was utterly and fully devastated. That's just friends, family, and business, I guess.

Dad and I used to hang out together before dark, golfing, rollerblading, shooting hoops; then we'd run our hands down the feed troughs to encourage the chickens to eat when the sun went down. Suddenly, I found myself alone at dusk. He stopped joining me. I knew something had changed, but I didn't have the words to describe it.

About eight months into the breakdown, my dad couldn't sleep. He just lay in bed crying. My mom took him to a doctor hoping something could help him cope. Without understanding what was going on in my dad's brain, the doctor prescribed anti-anxiety medication to help him sleep. He popped them like candy, taking as many as he could so he could fall asleep and escape the pain he felt deep within his core. It was a huge mistake. We were at a loss of what to do, and we didn't know it was about to get much worse.

With no end to my dad's lethargy and dissociation in sight, my mom started to take my dad to every healer, pastor, therapist, psychiatrist, and guru imaginable. She had him try acupuncture, mindful meditation, counseling, took him to see more doctors and pastors, brewed strange eastern medicine tea, but nothing alleviated his symptoms. It took six years before a Christian therapist said that he couldn't help my dad and referred him to a psychiatrist named Dr. Erso.

"You have severe depression," Dr. Erso told my dad. He explained what depression was, how it's a cycle that goes on in your brain. He told my dad that most patients feel bad about feeling bad and that it was okay not to feel okay.

"Depression is basically an injury to the brain. It takes a long time to heal," he said. My dad sat there, processing the information.

"Have you made any major financial decisions since the depression began?" Dr. Erso asked.

"Yes," my dad said, his eyes lowered. You could see the pain in his face, and guilt, and general bad feelings knowing our family was facing financial ruin. I can only imagine what it actually was like for him, sitting there, wishing he had found this doctor years earlier.

"That's okay. It is in the past. You cannot be concerned with decisions you made in the past. Our goal is to get you as comfortable as possible, with the correct medication and therapy, so your brain can heal. You just have to think about your future," he said.

He was the first truly caring and properly trained physician who had the experience to actually explain depression to our family in a way we understood. Not only did it help our family, but the treatment gave my dad a glimmer of hope. Dr. Erso took away the stigma and taught us the facts about this sinister illness.

I wish I could say my dad returned to his old self with the medication and therapy helped my dad get back to his old self, but that is far from the truth. The depression and anti-anxiety medication led Dad down a free fall path to self-medication and destruction. When he ran out of his "anxiety" pills, he'd have people go to Mexico, about two and a half hours away, to fetch him more. For an addict that didn't want people to know or see what they were doing, Mexico was the perfect place to find a fix at a low price. It was telling that our tight-knit Christian community couldn't help us with the financial disaster we were facing, but someone out there, for the right price, was always willing to run down to Mexico to fetch Dad more pills. It was frustrating and we, as a family, felt helpless. If that plan failed, he turned to alcohol. He was desperate to numb the pain, the rejection, and most of all, the crushing feeling of failure. He wanted to shut the world out and would stop at nothing to do it.

If the vices ran dry, my dad checked into rehab. He learned this after his inaugural hospitalization for withdrawal when he got violently ill. The very first time he did this, he agreed to attend some sort of treatment. We were hopeful. Maybe he'd get the structured assistance he desperately needed with more professionals. He'd plow through withdrawal, with minimal issues because he was provided medication to calm his body, as he purged the numbing toxins. Upon his release, he ran right back into the comforting and familiar arms of the prescribed medication and alcohol to numb the cycle of feeling down, low, and anxious. The cycle repeated itself about every six months, and he'd check into rehab again. This happened at least eight times over 12 years.

It was frustrating, but I didn't have time to be angry at him. As much as I shut my emotions off, seeing my dad, the most fun person ever who had the brightest spark for life, lose that vitality and become the most miserable and sad person was the most heavy and heartbreaking thing that I had ever witnessed. I felt horrible for him. I realized that nothing lasts; nothing remains the same.

This person did not feel like my dad, the steadfast provider who wanted nothing but to fill our lives with joy and smiles. It wasn't always this way. My brother, sister, and I had a magical childhood filled with everything we could ever want. Our lives were full of fun family vacations and quality time spent together. We could afford anything we wanted or needed. But everything changed as my dad's depression spiraled. My mom, meanwhile, took a job as a waitress to put food on the table. Now that we were dirt poor and borderline destitute, learning how much things cost was eye opening.

Our family never asked for handouts, but it was obvious we were in dire straits. Yet, our church community believed in pride and perseverance. It was against the grain to complain and admit fault, and many thought depression was sadness, something you could simply "snap out of." The people around us didn't consider it a real disease. It wasn't viewed as something tangible and real.

*   *   *

My doctors thought my new routine of living my dream in D.C. was causing the low blood sugars. I had no choice but to take them at their word. Since I couldn't figure out if there was another test or treatment for which I should be advocating, I thanked them and got ready for my next adventure.

Before jumping back into the trenches, my friends suggested we go on an end-of-year celebration cruise to Bermuda and the Bahamas, because three of them were graduating. It had been a while since I had gone on a "real" vacation. I happily bought a ticket and joined in on the fun. It helped that I also had some money saved from working at a hotel; my student loans covered much of my law school expenses. I didn't have any income in D.C., but I had a credit card for emergencies. The cruise was too inexpensive not to go for nine days and we didn't have to fly. We took the train to Baltimore and a taxi to the port.

Code Blue

We boarded the cruise ship in Baltimore, Maryland. This would be my first time going to the Caribbean. Our days on the cruise mirrored our weekends in D.C. with fun, laughter, adventure, and camaraderie. Sometimes my friends would do their own thing during the day, but we'd all come together and eat as a group at night. The pink sand beach in Bermuda was a breathtaking sight. Swimming in the waves with brightly colored fish and man o' war jellyfish was simply amazing to experience.

I found locals and fellow tourists who were willing to play three-on-three basketball for a few hours, and we had the time of our lives. One of my friends loved to sing karaoke, so we'd hang out and watch him try to woo the crowd. All of us tried to play the daily lottery, and it was a fun thing to look forward to each day, but we never won. Throughout the day, we would hear codes across the ship's intercom, such as code green, code PVI, code 30-30, etc. We made a game out of guessing what the different codes meant. In addition to our daily lottery struggles, the codes became an inside joke with our group.

As the end of the cruise was approaching, various specials started popping up on the boat. We had two days to fill as we traveled back to Baltimore from the Bahamas. At this point, I had done just about every single thing you could do on a cruise. I was still having fun, but was looking for something different to do. I found an advertisement for a special on 60-minute massages and thought that would be a nice way to complete my vacation experience. On our last day on the water, I booked a late afternoon massage for 5:00 p.m. We had reservations later that evening at the fancy steakhouse, and I wanted to make sure I had time to get ready for our final cruise dinner celebration.

After a brief introduction with the massage therapist, a nice woman with an English accent, I laid down on the massage table and closed my eyes, ready for an hour of relaxation before returning to the hectic hustle and bustle of D.C. life. But that's not what I got.

"I got a read!" someone shouted.

My eyes shot open as pain radiated through my chest. I gasped for air, crying out in pain and total confusion, as four people peered down at me, asking me a million questions at once.

What is happening? I thought to myself, sobbing. A woman was holding my head and kept telling me that everything was okay. Just try to remain calm.

The last thing I remembered was laying down on the massage table. From what I could tell, I was still on the massage table. There was a lot of commotion going on around me and I had no clue what was going on. Feeling extremely panicky, I wondered why my chest hurt so much?

Someone kept trying to stick my left hand with something sharp, a needle or maybe an IV. I couldn't move. I laid there, tears streaming down my face, confused, and hoping the woman holding my head would explain what was going on. Another person gave me a sip of something sweet that tasted like sugar water. Within a few moments, I started to feel more aware and could begin to respond to all their questions.

"What are you doing to me?" I asked.

All at once the questions stopped. An older man spoke up in an authoritative voice, "I was just about to pronounce you dead."

"What do you..." was all I could say. I wondered if I had a low blood sugar episode.

"I told them you're a diabetic," a familiar voice in the distance said. "I'm glad you're alright, man."

It was my trusted law school friend who always had my back. I started to piece things together with what little information I had. Once I was coherent enough to answer questions, confirm I was not on drugs and had not been drinking alcohol, I explained it could be my hypoglycemia. The medical team put me on a gurney and wheeled me from the back of the ship, where the spa was located, to the middle of the ship where the elevators were. I was rolled all the way to the bow where the medical center was located. Along the way, I had people gawking at me with judgment smeared across their faces. I was extremely embarrassed. *How did I get into this situation without being aware of anything,* I thought?

"At some point during your massage, you passed out. We have no idea how long you were out for," the doctor who was going to declare me dead said. "You weren't breathing and did not have a heartbeat when we got here. We shocked you twice with the defibrillator. It didn't work."

"Your friend here showed up and was yelling that you're a type 1 diabetic, probably having a low blood sugar event. I'll be honest, we gave him a hard time because we were trying to save your life, but when he said you were suffering from a low blood sugar, we gave you a dose of glucagon and tried the defibrillator one more time," the doctor explained.

"How long was I out for?" I asked the doctor.

"We don't know for sure, but we have it recorded here that you did not have a heartbeat for at least eight minutes. I've never seen anything like this before. You must have someone looking out for you."

Shit.

I sat in a hospital bed in the medical clinic while the team kept checking my vitals and blood sugar. One of the medical staff said someone was in the waiting room asking if they could see me, and I told her to let them back. My friend, the one who just went out of his way to help, stood in the corner of the room, concerned, yet relieved. The doctor scribbled notes and took my information down. He gave me instructions to go directly to my doctor when I got to shore because something was wrong, and it clearly needed to be addressed. He also said I needed to go back to my room and rest and relax for the rest of the night because I had been through a lot. He didn't want me to end up back in the infirmary. After a few hours, I was finally allowed to leave. They wheeled me to my room and provided the direct line to the medical center. I thanked them, glad it was over.

"I heard the code and I remembered you went to get a massage," my friend told me. "I had a feeling it was you."

"Thank you! I think you seriously saved my life," I told him. "I had my medical alert bracelet on. I told them I was diabetic, but apparently they didn't take that information seriously. If you hadn't said anything, I probably would have died in the most relaxing way possible; but, all jokes aside, I owe you my life."

He brushed it off like it was no big deal, but I could never thank him enough.

It wasn't the first time my medical ID was ignored.

I have no idea how or why I survived. The ship hit me with a hefty medical bill that I had to put on my credit card because I wasn't prepared to spend thousands of dollars on a medical emergency. I would find out later that insurance didn't cover it because I was in "international waters." Before I got ready to go see my friends and enjoy the rest of the last night on the ship, there was something I knew I had to do. The massage therapist probably thought she killed me, so I returned to the spa.

"Hi," I said, as I knocked gingerly on the closed door with a closed sign dangling on the outside. The massage staff appeared to be having a meeting, most likely about what happened to me, sadly.

"You guys had nothing to do with this," I told them. "I have a disease and I'm not in control of it." I tried my best to explain.

My massage therapist started to cry.

"I'm so sorry this happened on your watch," I told her.

She walked over to me, looking me up and down as if she didn't believe I was truly alive.

"Do you know what happened?" I asked her, since the medical staff didn't really give me details leading up to their intervention.

"You were really quiet after the first 15 minutes," she said, still sobbing. "You were talkative at first and asked where I was from and told me why you were on the vacation, then you went quiet. I thought you didn't want to talk anymore. When we were done, I told you to get dressed and you didn't move, so I left for a few minutes thinking you needed more time. I knocked on the door and you didn't answer. I knocked again and opened the door and you were just lying there. I walked over to wake you because I thought you might be sleeping, but you didn't move. You looked dead. That's when I called the emergency responders."

"Once again, I am so sorry this happened. This is 100 percent my fault. It's related to my diabetes, but I promise you had nothing to do with it," I repeated.

I left her the biggest tip I possibly could. Deep down I knew I had traumatized her, and there wasn't a damn thing I could do to take that back.

"Are you okay?" my friends asked when I finally met back up with them.

At this time, I was finally mentally back with it. I missed the dinner reservation and felt horrible because they canceled it once they heard I had an emergency. I felt fine...as fine as you can feel after a near death situation. My attitude was still about having the time of my life and not letting something interfere with that. Maybe I was so relaxed my body just wanted to stop fighting for a bit. I made a few jokes about it to ease the tension and told them not to worry. The big joke was that we learned what one of the codes really meant—code blue meant emergency. And all my friends laughed because I got to experience that one first hand. The remainder of the night went by without incident.

When we returned to Baltimore, I called my endocrinologist to explain what had happened. This was serious. Also, it was really embarrassing to be found in a state like that. Even if it was my reality, my doctors needed to know. And, this was now impacting other people.

"You need to eat more," she told me. "Did you eat protein and complex carbohydrates or a graham cracker before the massage?" Again, I felt patronized. I didn't eat the graham cracker, but I was damn sure I ate something. I ate plenty on the ship. I didn't know what to think. What I did know is that I was grateful for everyone on that ship who saved my life and didn't give up on me despite my being dead for at least eight minutes. Also, I'm so glad my friend advocated for me in my time of need.

Two days later, my State Department internship started. I walked into the main building. It was large, dull white, and quite underwhelming. The offices, rooms, hallways, bathrooms, elevators, and everything else were very small. They were smaller than you would imagine for such a large and powerful governmental organization. I expected far more grandeur but at the end of the day, it's a building that people work in. I got lost a few times trying to find specific rooms with more than 1,000 other interns, trying to get an ID. This went on every day for a week as the new interns were processed. My orientation went smoothly and I learned that I would be working in Arlington, Virginia, just outside D.C., across the Potomac River. I learned my security protocols, how'd I use my ID to get into buildings, and what stop I'd need to get off on the Metro. On my first day, I couldn't stay awake during one of the presentations. Despite my interest in what was being said, my head kept bobbing. One of the staff members talked to me afterwards and said I'd have to return to listen to the presentation again, as it was a matter of 'national security,' and then I would need to sign that I attended. *How humiliating! Why was this happening?*

I still felt that fiery passion and purpose coursing through my veins for the work that I was doing. I hadn't told my parents about the cruise incident. I hoped it would be an isolated event, and I didn't want to worry them. Instead, I dove headfirst into the rare opportunity I had earned and wished the blood sugar would sort itself out like my doctors said it would.

Somehow, though, I knew that wasn't going to be the case.

CHAPTER 6

The Metro Incident

Even though it was a rough first day of orientation with my blood sugars trying to knock me down, I had it in my mind that nothing was going to stop me. I was officially a legal intern with the State Department. Just the task of procuring my security clearance took more than six months. That was a testament to how prestigious this opportunity was. Every morning when I woke up, I was excited and filled with gratitude. I'd get dressed, pack my tan canvas bag with plenty of Mentos and Gatorade and snacks, and venture to the Metro, eagerly anticipating my workday.

The memory of my code blue on that cruise remained nestled in the corner of my mind. Every doctor lacked a diagnosis and the only medical advice that was provided by the professionals was to eat more often. For my own personal wellbeing, I did. A lot. But the low blood sugars continued. In fact, they were intensifying. My body was shutting down more often and it was ten times worse when

I was alone without someone to keep an eye on me. The exhaustion and fatigue were starting to get to me, but I refused to give in. My body would not ruin this once-in-a-lifetime opportunity for me.

At the start of my internship, I did a lot of research. It was absolutely fascinating. I had a small cubicle surrounded by many other small cubicles. Boring, I know, but every aspect of the job made me happy. I enjoyed using my badge to enter buildings, elevators, and floors. Most found the need to use their badge for everything a nuisance, but it reminded me of how fortunate I was for the opportunity to use it. It was proof of something I could never imagine myself to be a part of because it was too unbelievable. With each passing day, I began to see a future in D.C. for myself.

Even though I was an intern, I was a minuscule part of things much larger than myself and helping accomplish things that benefited people. Moreover, everyone I was around had the same goal. Maybe feeling that way is exactly what I needed. I wasn't overeating for comfort, I wasn't lost looking for a purpose, I wasn't bitter that my talents weren't being used. Everything was just perfect. Except for my low blood sugars. But, I separated that from the good that was happening in my life. I felt those lows were part of the territory of living with a chronic illness and hoped they would resolve. I had been on a journey for a taste of contentment and joy and happiness since the egg ranch debacle. It's interesting how the passions and excitement for my internship seemed to be influenced by what I experienced during my younger years.

From the ages of 16 to 21, I felt as if I had lived a full life already. I grew up way too fast in much too short of a time to realize what having a purpose or reason or proper expectation about life was all about. During my dad's depression, I handled business deals (which taught me a lot about people) and large amounts of money.

The Metro Incident

I think the ranch was my dad's purpose in our family. When the business failed, the life my dad built was stripped away with his sense of purpose. I looked at my dad and felt absolute sorrow and sadness that I could do nothing to help him. It just fed into my anger, bitterness, and resentment. I was never mad or upset at him. Once Dr. Erso explained what was going on, I understood his struggle. But the man who taught me how to golf, ride a bike, who let me put a delivery van in gear when I was five years old, who showed me the value of hard work and determination, was gone. I knew it. He knew it. The idea of getting better seemed bleak, if not impossible. I felt in some ways, he'd be better off if he were dead. Then, at least he'd be free. He would be at peace. Back then, that is all I wanted for him - to not hurt any more.

When I was 21, we still had our local accounts and our egg store. We were still packing eggs and doing everything that we could to keep up with the accounts. And I mean everything. Keeping a small egg ranch was fine, we could pay our bills and our employees, but it just wasn't enough to support a family of five. We had utility bills, grocery bills, medical bills, etc. My mom worked tirelessly at her job at a restaurant. I found work with UPS and a health food store in addition to the ranch. We got by, enough so we weren't on the streets, but barely. However, I needed more in life. I craved purpose.

*   *   *

I caught a glimpse of purpose in 2004 when a friend invited me to go with him to Mexico on a mission trip. He was going with our church's Bible study group. At that point in my life, I hadn't taken a trip in years—probably since that fateful one to Michigan. I decided to go and see what it was all about. I packed all the necessities: clothes, toiletries, and diabetic supplies and headed to Mexico with about 20 volunteers.

It was exactly that kind of break I needed. I spent four days working on various projects the local church had set up for us. We helped repair structural damage at impoverished orphanages. We dug a hole in the ground so the community could build a bathroom. We constructed buildings, including a house. We replaced water pipes. We helped to feed and entertained the locals who met at the church each evening for their sustenance, after which we would gather together to process the day and all we had witnessed. I was in awe. During my magical childhood, I saw many things and encountered many people, but I was absolutely blown away by the poverty and living conditions. I mean, the people had nothing.

If a local was fortunate enough to live near a power line, everyone would run a wire to the line and somehow split into it. Sewage ran down the streets and into nearby water. Houses lacked foundations, so most people lived on dirt. I didn't understand how they earned money, how they paid for shelter, food, and clothes, or how they got around. What would happen if there was an emergency? How would it be handled if one of their children had Diabetes like me? But, despite living in poverty, they were SO full of joy. I had way more stuff than they did, even though I thought I had nothing because of all we had lost. I felt I could not find joy, and yet, here in Mexico, were people with literally next to nothing, grinning from ear to ear and enjoying the company of one another.

Kids ran around playing with oblivious innocence. This reminded me of my younger siblings, since Mom and I tried hard to shelter them from the difficulties happening to our family. Elders sat outside with neighbors, sharing stories and enjoying the sun. I felt a bit of resentment at their easy camaraderie with family, friends, and strangers alike; and I could not help but think most of my own elders were severely lacking in comparison. I marveled at the simplicity the community enjoyed. Witnessing their lives and what they found value in made me realize something important. I wanted to be a part of it and I wanted to help make their lives better. Maybe I could go help people find new water sources or make sure kids weren't freezing to death at night or help get medical, specifically diabetic, supplies where they were needed. For the first time in my life, I saw a future outside of the egg ranch.

That trip was life changing in a way, because it led me to discover and be accepted at Bible College, a two-year secondary program where I could take classes and prepare for a life of mission and service. It seemed like a natural fit for someone who grew up in a Dutch Reform community, had attended Christian schools his whole life, and was looking for something more.

*   *   *

I sat in my cubicle, behind my computer, researching international law. My juice and backup low blood sugar snacks sat readily in the cabinet above my desk. I felt safe. I was happy. I was accepted to a prestigious internship, I found something I never thought would be possible. It gave me meaning and provided me purpose. It was something greater than myself. I felt like my future was limitless and I was finally where I was meant to be. I wanted to feel like this for the rest of my life.

Each evening as the sun started to set on the Potomac River, I would pack up my work papers and things before heading out to the Metro to go home. I liked to use my phone to track my steps and the distance I traveled, so I knew that each day I walked about 10 miles, in addition to my time on the Metro. I had always been active, so I never really noticed just how far I traveled on foot. This probably had a lot to do with the hustle and bustle of the city, combined with the music and podcasts on my headphones, making my walks easy and enjoyable. The only thing that slowed me down was my recovery after a low blood sugar. Otherwise, I would usually be buzzing with energy from my day and all the neat things I got to be a part of.

One evening after a long day of meetings, research, and little tasks in between, I said goodnight to my colleagues as I headed out to the Metro. When I boarded the train, I picked an empty seat in the front of the car. I typically didn't sit on the metro or go to the front because it was so busy. It was easier to maneuver around people in the mid to back section of the cars and stand. However, I sat there quietly, reflecting on my day, and planning what I'd have for dinner once I got home.

Screech!

The train stopped on the tracks and startled me awake. I must have nodded off between stops. I looked around to realize I was seven stops from where I needed to be. I frantically looked around the train. I was the only one there. *How was that possible? It was in the heat of the evening commute. Did the train break down?*

I reached into my pocket and pulled out my phone. It read 12:00 a.m. I had been sitting in the same spot for six hours. SIX HOURS! The train wasn't moving. Within minutes a conductor would do a sweep of the cars, making sure everyone was off the train for the night. It was the end of the line. I was bewildered. The last thing I remembered was sitting down in that empty seat. It was like the cruise ship all over again, except this time there were no terrified massage therapists or defibrillators.

I gathered my things and gingerly exited the Metro in absolute confusion, working on autopilot. It was a ghost town. As I headed for the street level, my phone started buzzing rapidly. I had missed many calls and messages. I put the phone back in my pocket because I needed to do two things before anything else. One: I needed to find food. Two: I needed to figure out where I was and exactly how far I was from home. I walked around the block and found a pizza shop that happened to be open. Quickly, I ordered a pepperoni pizza and asked for a drink cup while my pizza was baking, so I could get some sugary liquid in my system before paying. My Gatorade was in my bag, but I wasn't thinking clearly at that point. I was in shock.

It turned out that I was five miles from home. Normally that distance would be an easy feat for me, but tonight was different. I was shaken up from passing out on the Metro and low on energy. It was late, and I didn't know how long pizza and Coke would sustain me. For all I knew, another low blood sugar could strike at any time. Then what? Would I just pass out on the streets of D.C. and hope I'd be found? Instead, I requested an Uber to take me home as I replayed the scene over and over in my mind. I was out for six whole hours. As far as I know, no one tried to wake me. As I sat in the back seat of the Uber, I surveyed my belongings. Nothing was taken. I usually was never fearful of theft or robbery in the city, even though it was common, but I was sure I had made an excellent target for crime, given my comatose state. I sighed, relieved everything was accounted for (including my security badge). Once I got home, I ate, showered, and went to bed. My blood sugar was really getting out of hand and it was scary. I didn't know what else I could change to stop the lows from happening so randomly.

For the week after the Metro incident, I did what I do best: I managed. I ate continuously. Even with a CGM, I checked my blood sugar hourly, and also made sure I was rarely alone. That last part was tough, but I knew I needed my coworkers to keep a watchful eye on me. Having to be vulnerable for survival's sake, I explained to two coworkers that I was a diabetic and that I have low blood sugar episodes at random times. I told them that an episode makes me look pale, sweaty, or out of it, like I'm drunk, and they should tell me to drink juice or call 911 if they ever find me in that state. They agreed to check on me no matter what and that helped me feel safer. They didn't have any obligation to take on any responsibility for me, but they did so willingly. I showed them where my stash of food and sugary drinks were in my cubicle. I needed their help to stay conscious, and my colleagues stepped up.

I thought I had things somewhat under control since I had not randomly passed out, that I could recall, in two weeks. My boss, the department director, asked that I put together a presentation for the department based on the work I had been doing. I flicked through my slides and explained the data with expert precision until I noticed one of my colleagues giving me a funny look as they asked me a question.

"Brandon, sit down. Sit down," they said. I listened. "Drink this," someone else said, handing me a bottle of my orange Gatorade. As the sugar flooded my body, my head started to clear. "What happened?" I asked, while everyone looked at me in shock.

"All of the sudden you lost all the color in your face, started sweating, and talking nonsense. It was like gibberish or a whole different language," my colleague commented, a look of worry and confusion plastered across her face.

"I am SO SORRY!" I said. "This is one of my low blood sugar episodes."

My director ended the meeting right then and there. We were all sent back to our work areas. I was embarrassed once again.

That afternoon, my director called me into her office to discuss what had occurred. I couldn't believe that my low blood sugars were now impacting my work. It wasn't fair to put someone in the position of being responsible for me or for them to see me in such a vulnerable state. Having low blood sugar is equivalent to me being at my worst. As I walked to my director's office, I thought, *this is it; I'm going to be asked to pack up my stuff, go home, and never come back.*

"Are you okay?" she asked ever so gently.

"Yes, I am so sorry. I let you down by not finishing my presentation and having a low blood sugar episode," I quickly replied.

"Give me an example of what happens to you during these episodes," she said.

I told her about the cruise and the Metro incident. She was shocked. "I know this is not your fault and it sounds like you're doing everything right, but it keeps happening. Brandon, this is dangerous stuff. You could have been mugged or killed on the Metro," she told me with a voice of compassion rather than a reprimanding tone.

"What can we do to help you?"

Everyone in D.C. had been nothing but kind and supportive, yet I still found myself surprised that the director would go to great lengths to keep me on board. D.C. was a cutthroat environment. If you showed any signs of weakness, there were tons of young, eager, and able-bodied interns ready to take your place in a second. The fact that my director really cared about me meant more than I realized.

"What options are there for someone who can't know or control when they are having low blood sugar?" she asked, reframing her question before I could say there was nothing anyone could do but keep an eye on me.

"Well, there is a diabetic alert option. A service dog. They cost a fortune and the wait period to secure one is a minimum of five years," I told her. "The other option is a pancreas transplant, but the doctors tell me that I'm too healthy for one."

"We're getting you that dog," she said matter-of-factly.

CHAPTER 7

Unexpected Friends

From that day forward, my director gave me an hour each day (usually my lunch break) to make calls and conduct research to find a diabetic alert dog. She also established a system where I'd need to text when I got home so she knew I was safe. If I didn't respond in a certain amount of time, she'd call the Metro police or emergency services to search for me, since she knew the route I took home. It wasn't a surefire plan, but it at least meant someone was keeping tabs on me when I was "alone" and not with friends or colleagues.

Each day, I made numerous calls to diabetic alert dog trainers and organizations. The prices were astronomical. Some went for $10,000 and some went for $50,000. All of the dogs had wait lists of several years before they could be placed with an owner, but I didn't give up. I knew I needed this to live. My director checked in on my findings as often as she checked in on my actual internship work. She was invested in me and my needs and made suggestions of places to contact when I came up empty.

Finally, after what seemed like 200 messages and voicemails that were never returned, I connected with a lady who lived in northern California. She was training her last set of diabetic alert dogs and had more than 30 years of experience in the training field. I told her I was from California and explained my dire situation to her. As an act of good faith (and perhaps a "swan song" of her retirement), she told me she'd have a dog ready for me. She had been saving him for the adult program where he'd be trained to open doors, bring juice or glucose tablets to the owner, and call the emergency line. Since the adult program takes a year and a half to train the service animal, she had not accepted any deposits on him yet. This meant no wait list!

The dog had completed his first set of training. He could go onto an advanced stage where he'd be trained to dial 911 in the event of an emergency, but the trainer feared I needed the alert dog immediately. This dog would normally go for $40,000. If I could pick him up in a month, I could have him for $10,000, since he wouldn't be going through the advanced training. He was six months old. I was so grateful. After so many setbacks and no's in the realm of diabetic alert service dogs, someone threw me a lifeline and said yes.

However, I didn't have $10,000 to pay for the dog. How was I going to come up with that kind of money in such a short amount of time? I called my grandma, on my Mom's side, and explained what was going on and she sent the money immediately. I couldn't believe it. In my state of absolute need, I was given another green light, a yes, a go, and provided help. That was not what my experiences with extended family had prepared me for. I didn't know how to feel about it, but knew that I was going to get help that I absolutely needed.

With six weeks left in my internship, I moved into an office with a coworker who would keep an eye on me and make sure I wouldn't pass out. She really had my back and made sure I was okay each day. Without her caring kindness, generosity, and friendship, I would not have been able to finish. It was different, having friends who had my back.

The trainer sent me pictures of the dog, which I showed all my friends and family. Due to some timing issues, I knew I'd have to end my internship early to pick him up right away, before my six weeks were up. Not wanting to end my internship early, I decided I'd wait until the internship ended. My director agreed. That was the best decision. There would be a chance I wouldn't get full credit for my internship if I left early, even to get this lifesaving dog.

Somehow, I made it through those six weeks without passing out completely or causing alarm. I thank my boss and coworker for that. I finished the semester strong knowing I had health stuff to figure out, but was going to be back in D.C. working and living my best life in no time. The morning after my last day, I flew to California, my mom picked me up from the airport, and we began the nine-hour drive to northern California to pick up the dog. My mind was racing. What was this going to look like? Was it going to be successful or an utter failure? A lot of time, energy, and money were invested to reach this point and my life depended on him being a successful diabetic alert dog. And, time was of the essence. This required a quick turnaround. My next semester of law school was days away.

I was tired, nervous, and excited. As we drove up the 5 Freeway, a familiar road, my exhausted mind began to recall the first time I truly stepped out of my comfort zone.

*   *   *

The first time "away" from home was when I attended Bible College, but it was close to the ranch. I was still able to work and maintain our accounts. Also, it was very inexpensive to attend, a plus for someone in my financial situation. This would be the first time that I truly did something for myself.

Back then, I was so bitter and angry and trying to figure everything out. Blow after blow, lawsuit after lawsuit, unpaid bill after unpaid bill, it all contributed to the walls I built around myself. I needed to do something to get me away from it all. I needed something that would allow me time to process, recharge, and learn a new skill. Furthermore, I needed to find something that would bring purpose and joy back into my life.

I was three years out of high school and eligible, due to working and quitting employment from UPS, for 18 months of COBRA health insurance, which would help me manage my diabetes and afford the supplies. At the time, one bottle of insulin cost upwards of $300 (and still does today), and I needed multiple bottles per month. Test strips were $1 a strip and I had to test my blood 5-7 times a day. Insurance companies could, at the time, deny coverage if you had a pre-existing condition, so it was important I kept some coverage. This was before the Affordable Care Act. If you couldn't be insured, it was an impossible situation to live with a chronic illness without help to cover costs.

My inaugural days at Bible College were about as eye opening as Mexico. The campus was stunningly beautiful—an old resort built around natural hot springs. Every original building on the property was preserved. Tall, California-esq fan palm trees outlined the freshly paved gated entrance. It was like stepping into another world, kind of like going to Disneyland. New buildings also had been built over the years including a few chapels, and a conference center for meetings.

In addition, the college was full of homeschooled kids, and though I felt old compared to most of them, I did make a few friends, both in and out of classes. We spent Tuesday evenings at a coffee shop playing board games. I felt kind of normal, but my friendships were not that deep. I was still jaded, guarded, and had trouble trusting others. My friends were just people I hung out with. We did fun things together, but I never opened myself up to them. I didn't want people to know where I came from or what my family was going through. It wasn't anyone's business anyway.

I was beginning to discover who I really was with each passing day. Every semester, each student was required to "participate" in an M-99. It was eight hours a week of "labor" around the college, disguised as a service class called M-99. Regardless, I thrived in my first semester assignment: landscaping. It was right in my wheelhouse, having perfected my lawn mowing cut lines on the ranch. For the second semester, I was chosen to be a Teaching Assistant (TA). When I got word of my assignment, I was genuinely offended. Why had I been taken away from what I found joy in doing? I had a part in maintaining the beauty of campus, and knew I was doing a good job with that assignment.

The problem, and I use the word "problem" ironically, was that I had proven myself as responsible, reliable, and organized based on my zero absences, communications with instructors and TAs, and getting to know staff around campus. As a TA, I made sure my instructors had everything they needed: water bottles, attendance sheets, grading inputted, announcements, make-up alerts written, you name it. I made sure all students signed in before the start of class and tracked down anyone who was absent. My knack for these administrative tasks was probably born out of my years running the ranch.

I learned I could accomplish all of my TA duties in about two hours. The rest of my eight hours was spent in the TA office asking for extra things to do to fulfill my obligations. It did not go unnoticed. Professors started sending students to me for some extra help. Little did I know, I would come to enjoy teaching. I hated school, but I liked helping others understand. Some students actually said they would have failed if I hadn't helped them, and that validation felt good. I found fulfillment being able to help somebody understand something they couldn't.

I began to entertain the possibility of becoming a teacher instead of a missionary. Teaching would provide health insurance, which was a consideration every time I thought about my future. I had some dissenting beliefs from what was being taught, but teaching seemed like a way for me to have purpose, make a difference, and help people. It felt natural.

No one at school knew about my life on the ranch or what had happened with my family. The walls I built were too high. With knowledge comes power and if someone knew too much about me, they might use it against me somehow. It wasn't worth the risk to let anyone in.

While I was there, I was still trying my best to salvage the ranch and attend school. One afternoon, I was in the egg room at the ranch finishing up for the day. I heard a car pull up to the side of the building. I thought that was unusual, since most people stopped at the store and then tried to find my dad. I brushed my hands on my pants and walked outside to see who it was. A nicely dressed man exited his Mercedes and began to walk toward me. Great. Another prospective buyer, I thought. They seemed to be coming out of the woodwork.

"Hello," he said and introduced himself. "I'm interested in buying this property." *Get in line*, was my first thought.

"Could you give your dad my information?"

As if on autopilot, I reached out my hand to snatch the business card from his. I was about to return to my work when he stopped me.

"I know how much you guys owe, and I can help you with a plan to get rid of your debt and start fresh," he said.

That caught my attention. Most prospective buyers touted arbitrary dollar figures. "If you can make me a deal right now, I'll buy this property for X amount of dollars in cash," they would say. I'd relay this information to my dad, who always declined. He wasn't ready to sell. The egg ranch was a source of pride for him. It was his life's work. Also, in his depressed state, he thought it was the only source of income we had to support the family. He didn't understand it was actually costing us, or that my mom and I supported the family with our side jobs.

The guy in the Mercedes was 100 percent legitimate. He called back and said he wanted to get us an attorney to settle our financial matters. Turns out he wasn't another greedy real estate broker. Instead, he was a housing developer and wanted to develop a shopping center or housing on our property. Since everyone had to drive past the egg ranch to get into town, our land was the perfect location for a new development. Mom and I finally agreed to let him meet Dad. We didn't know what would come of the meeting, but we insisted Dad hear the guy out. This guy wasn't like the rest, and we hoped Dad would see that, too, even through the murky waters of his illness.

"I can see you are depressed," the Mercedes guy said to my dad when he finally agreed to meet. "We're going to do this right. I'm going to help your family get out of this financial hole and be transparent along the way."

We owed money to banks, feed companies, the egg boxing company, the list went on and on. We couldn't afford to pay all of our bills. The investments my dad had made during his depression had all tanked. It was time to sell if we wanted to survive. Finally, my dad conceded. He and my mom worked with the attorney to get to a place where they could walk away debt free. We sold every piece of equipment and every piece of property outside the ranch. We sold the ranch itself. My parents were able to walk away with nothing but a zero balance of debt. It was finally over. It was a relief. Of course, it was also sad; it was the end of an era, but it was the only viable choice we had left. There was a lot of love on that land and countless memories. It was a great place to grow up and I'll never forget it.

With my future dreams of running the ranch officially extinguished, it was time for a change. I remember while in the TA office, I overheard the Registrar talk about another Christian college in Phoenix, Arizona that would transfer existing Bible College credits. If I applied and got in, I could get my bachelor's degree in two years and start to build a career in something. At that point, teaching history appealed to me the most. Missionary work was out of the question and so I knew I wanted to find another way to help people.

*   *   *

"We're about fifteen minutes away, Brandon," my mom said, breaking my reverie. "Should you call the trainer to let her know?"

"No, I'll just text her," I said.

Now that we were minutes away, the prospect of getting a diabetic alert dog was exciting. The ability to have a dog that was trained to alert me that my blood sugar was dropping—even before a blood test—could save my life. Moments later we reached our destination. My mom and I hopped out of the car as I prepared to meet my lifesaving creature. The trainer walked out of the house with the fluffiest, most stunningly adorable, and regal-looking animal I had ever seen. A Standard Goldendoodle, named Boone, he was so calm and happy with wavy, light brown fur and big brown eyes that just kind of looked into your heart. He was much bigger than I anticipated, at least 40 pounds and very tall.

The trainer taught me all the commands and how Boone works. The training is pretty intensive, but the way diabetic alert dogs are taught how to do their job is pretty amazing and ingenious. A person with low blood sugar sucks on a cotton ball, puts the cotton ball with the low blood sugar saliva in a glass jar, and freezes it. Once there are 20 cotton balls or so, they are sent to the trainer. No matter the person, all low blood sugars smell the same to dogs. The trainer then uses the cotton ball as the scent for the dog to recognize when a person is having a low blood sugar episode. After the dog is trained on the smell and knows how to alert the trainer, the dog gets a treat as positive reinforcement.

At random times, the trainer takes the jar out of the freezer, opens it, and puts it somewhere in the room. She carefully watches to make sure the dog senses the low blood sugar, catches the scent and alerts as per his training. I couldn't believe how extensive and meticulous the training was.

I'm Still Kickin'

When you're a diabetic and your blood sugar drops fast, studies show your body excretes cholesterol from the liver to stop the sugar molecules from being burned up in your body. This reaction produces a smell that dogs can sense. It's amazing!

The first time Boone alerted me, we were in training with him in a store. The trainer showed me how Boone always walked on the left, how he walked around a cart, and what happened when people came up to ask to pet him. (Spoiler alert: You say, "No, he is a service dog.") We were standing in an aisle when all of the sudden Boone turned to look at the trainer. He looked at me, looked at her, looked back at me, and started pawing my leg. He sensed the smell my saliva gave off, indicating a low blood sugar episode! I didn't see that one coming.

Boone was trained to constantly paw me until I drank juice or ate and gave him a treat. The treat is his way of knowing his job is done. After three days, Boone and I flew back to Phoenix. I was ready to start my life with this amazing, lifesaving creature. It happened to be Boone's first flight. He was tucked under my legs on the floor in the bulkhead at the front of the plane because it had the most leg room. Boone takes up more than one seat of floor space. All of the sudden, he got up and put his paw on my knee.

"What's going on, Boone?" I asked him, gently scratching his head. "It's okay." He continued to paw at my leg again and again. Hard. He was starting to make marks underneath my jeans. I thought he was anxious about the flight and then it hit me. OH! I am having a low blood sugar episode! I grabbed the Mentos out of my pocket and popped as many as I could, as quickly as I could, in my mouth.

Unfortunately, I didn't have any treats on me at the time, so I had to say "good boy" as earnestly as possible for Boone to understand he did his job. He looked at me with those concerned, almost human eyes before laying back down at my feet. Flights are usually diverted during medical emergencies. If I didn't have Boone, I probably would have passed out on the plane and who knows what would have happened?

As the plane touched down in Phoenix, I looked down at Boone, who was ready for a command. *Let's see how all this goes*, I thought. "Up, heel," I said to him with a smile. He stood up, proudly at the ready and stepped to my left side, like he'd been practicing his whole life. It had only been a few days, but already I felt a sense of security knowing Boone had my back. It was a huge relief as I prepared to tackle my final year of law school.

CHAPTER 8
A Different Animal

Growing up, my life revolved around taking care of animals. Chickens, goats, sheep, cows, exotic birds, and we always had a dog on the ranch. Now I had this lifesaving canine, Boone, who depended on me just as much as I depended on him. It was a whole new dynamic. He was not an ordinary dog, by any means. Life with Boone was an interesting transition, starting out. I had to get him special boots so his paws wouldn't burn on the hellacious Arizona asphalt which can reach upwards of 250 degrees. I always made sure he wore his vest, so people knew he was a service animal as a diabetic alert dog. He came with me wherever I went, so I had to be equipped with everything he might need on any given day.

Caring for Boone was never a burden, but it was certainly an adjustment. His trainer warned me about what life would be like with a service dog. "Everywhere you go people are going to ask to pet him," she told me. "You have to tell them no. And everywhere you go where dogs aren't conventionally allowed, people are going to say you can't bring him."

I knew the law, but she made sure to reiterate my rights to me before we parted ways. Whenever someone tries to tell me he is not allowed, I am to say, "He is a service animal." The federal law states he provides a service that I require for a disability. His service dog credentials are marked clearly on his vest. Legally, Boone was allowed to be with me at all times in public spaces. Still, most people just didn't get it.

If we went to a restaurant or café, the hostess always offered the patio to us first, saying, "Dogs are allowed on the patio only." Going to the grocery store? "I'm sorry, sir, dogs aren't allowed here." Time and time again, I had to patiently educate people on the law and nature of the service dog. I even had a card with the U.S. Service Dog Law printed on it. If I got significant push back, I could voluntarily present that card.

It was exhausting, but as a law student, I never gave up a fight. I knew I wasn't the only guy with a service animal and plenty of people encounter the same discriminatory ignorance. I felt a need to educate people about others who have service animals. Looking back, if I had Boone as a kid, I don't know if I would have the ability to stick up for myself as an adult. I never want kids to feel ostracized for having a service animal. It is so frustrating when you try to take your service dog with you to a location and are met with "you're so spoiled, you think you're special." It makes you want to scream, "No, I need this service animal to stay alive!" This was just a part of life now. However, there are times I wish I did have Boone when I was a kid. He would have saved me from so many low blood sugar episodes.

A Different Animal

There were occasions when I was questioned about my disability or the nature of Boone's service. That question is 100 percent illegal, but sometimes I gave in. Of course, I may have done it with a bit of snark if the situation allowed. I think people saw me and did not think I was disabled since I appeared to be able bodied. Not all disabilities are visible. Everyone is different.

According to the federal Americans with Disabilities Act and HIPAA privacy provisions, the only questions that can be asked about a service dog are: Is the dog a service animal required because of a disability, and what has the dog been trained to do? Those are legitimate questions, however under HIPAA, no one is required to disclose their disability. It's considered protected information. For me, it was a delicate balance. I needed to have Boone with me, but I didn't need to declare to the world that I was a diabetic with crushing low blood sugars who relied on Boone to save my life.

To answer the questions, I would legally respond with, "He is a trained service animal for my disability, and I am required to have him with me for my disability." Generally, people did not like that answer. Even though I answered their question, and legally, I didn't have to tell them about my disability, people are still nosy and often are wanting more specific information. It is sad to say that many individuals, restaurants, stores, bowling alleys, airlines, rideshare services, etc., sometimes have discriminatory attitudes towards people with disabilities—especially if there is a dog involved.

The good news was that I had Boone for my final year of law school. Boone became a celebrity at law school. He helped to initiate many conversations about Diabetes that would not have transpired otherwise, and he displayed the life-saving power of a service animal. Once the students and faculty realized what he did, people at school let Boone do his job uninterrupted. From August to October, life was pretty normal. Boone alerted me every time I had a low blood sugar (which was frequently). I went to class, wrote my papers, and made plans to take the bar exam. For the first time since the crazy low blood sugar episodes began, I felt like I didn't have to worry about my health as much. Sure, it was troubling to still have these symptoms, but at least with Boone, I wasn't passing out at random places. Still, I had many low blood sugars, but Boone alerted me the instant my blood sugar began dropping, even before my glucose monitor would catch it. With Boone by my side, I wasn't passing out at random.

The kidney stones, low blood sugars, Washington, D.C., and now Boone were all new things in my life. With each one, I had to learn how to adapt and move forward, embracing each change and the lessons offered along the way. As an adult, the first major life change I was faced with happened in Bible College. I discovered my zest for mission work was not what I expected and had faded. It was time to consider other possibilities.

*   *   *

Even with my TA service assignment responsibilities, I ended up having extra time on my hands. With this extra time, I tutored students who requested extra help. Turns out, I did well. Helping other students to understand how to write and complete assignments made me acknowledge another option for my future. I knew I could get my degree, become a teacher, and secure exceptional health insurance with a teaching job. I mean, that's what you hear about teaching jobs—that the benefits are awesome. Tutoring at Bible College had awakened a more practical sense of purpose within me. I finally discovered a liking for certain school subjects, mainly history and politics. Running a classroom would probably be akin to running the ranch. There were processes to follow and order to maintain, plus everyone works toward a goal (passing the class). It seemed like it could be a good fit for me.

On the day I received mail that would put me on an unexpected path, I was excited. It was rare for emotions to break through my walls, but lately those emotions had been positive. I opened it up and discovered some fantastic news. I had been accepted full-time at the Christian college in Phoenix, and it felt damn good to have another acceptance under my belt. Due to my financial circumstances, I was approved for the highest level of financial aid. With grants and student loans, I'd be able to afford room, board, books and of course, tuition. I packed up my necessities and set out for Phoenix, "flying the coop," for the first time.

I started school in January, halfway through the regular school year, so I was classified as a transfer student. Arizona was hot and dry. Outside of Phoenix, there wasn't much around. Sure, Arizona had plenty of natural wonders like Sedona and the Grand Canyon, but I had to plan a whole trip out to see those. It wasn't like the 30-minute drive to the ocean in California. The school itself was nothing like I thought it would be. The information packet contained beautiful pictures of a large campus with many students and classrooms. However, this was far from the truth. My new little Christian college had fewer students than the Bible College, and had one small building for classes. It certainly wasn't an old resort, nor did it have any beautiful plant life. Arizona had rocks instead of yards, which was hard for me to accept.

Since I was a transfer student, I discovered quite quickly that friend groups were already established. Nobody was very eager to welcome a newcomer into their friend group. It was amazing how strong those social circles had grown in just one semester.

It didn't bother me, though. I was there to earn my degree and move on. Plus, I didn't have to share any information about myself.

My new school was an adjustment; something I had to power through. When I arrived at my assigned dorm, I was surprised to see the room littered with trash and clothes. An unfamiliar stench wafted through the air. It was a stark contrast from the Bible College days where military-style bed checks were the norm. The egg ranch and our house were immaculate at all times. I wasn't accustomed to such a disorder. After a hasty introduction, I asked my roommates about the rules and was met with incredulous looks. Rules? What rules? It made me think about driving back to California and reassess my decision to move without visiting first.

My classes were small, and the coursework was relatively easy. It didn't take me long to figure out if I just did the readings and turned in the papers, I could get straight A's. Once I made the Dean's List, I thought, *I'm going to keep this up.* I decided that would be the goal I'd work toward: making straight A's in all of my classes. It was a tangible pursuit that allowed me to see my effort at the end of each grading period.

That first semester, however, was a total and complete blur, full of adjustments. From January until May, I just kept my head down and did my work. Despite my gentle pleas, my roommates were messy and preferred clutter, filth, and a lack of rules. It was a place to sleep, but nothing more. Dorm life in college was not for me. Needing money for my diabetic supplies and health insurance, I put in a few job applications, hoping to get work to pay for diabetic supplies, and I landed a position as a server at a restaurant nearby. They even offered health insurance and I could work as much as my class schedule would allow. Most of my checks went to diabetic supplies, and my car payment. If anything was left over, I sent it home to my mom.

Before the start of my second semester, I applied to be a Resident Assistant (RA) to get out of an unclean dorm room with unkind strangers. Management came naturally to me and working with people was a skill I cultivated from my years on the ranch. Luckily, I was offered an RA position. Due to my age and experience, I was assigned the more challenging floor of students. All floors generally had two RAs, but I would be managing my floor all on my own. The regulator in me lit up. I craved order and I wanted to fix what I viewed as a broken system. I didn't assume these kids were bad. I treated everyone equally and approached my residents with a clean slate and clear expectations.

Each day I would talk to the residents. I'd ask them how they were doing or how their history exam went. I'd ask about their basketball or soccer games and sometimes I'd even go to their games. If the resident was a music major, I'd make an attempt to attend their recitals. I made a point to support each and every student in their personal endeavors. With rules and a personal approach, my floor of "challenging" students became a well-structured, obedient residential floor with happy and successful college students.

In return for my increased responsibility as an RA, my room and board and cafeteria privileges were provided at no cost to me. Rather than share a room with a bunch of unruly strangers, I had a private mini-apartment with a small bedroom, a living room area with a large TV, and best of all, my own kitchen. I let my residents come in and cook whenever they pleased. I also hosted movie and game nights, where we'd order a pizza or cook a meal together and hang out in my living area.

As time went on, I made a few friends. Like Bible College, my friendships weren't that deep. I didn't talk about my life outside of college. People who got to know me picked up on the fact that I was a private person. Instead of prying or trying to get into my head, my friends were happy hanging out and doing fun things together. On the occasions they did ask me something deep about myself, all I had to do to deflect was to ask them a question about themselves. Nine times out of ten, they would happily answer and go back to talking about themselves. I did this often. The egg ranch, my dad's depression, the betrayal by family, friends, investors, and people in the church...all of it was my personal business. By revealing any of it, I believed I'd open myself up to vulnerability and people might use that information against me and somehow, someway take advantage. I couldn't allow myself to trust anyone.

Instead, I maintained a strong facade. It wasn't hard. My emotions were shut down like a cemented pipeline, deep underground, for no one to find. Yes, I had an empathic heart for my residents and fostered meaningful connections, but I did not internalize those relationships. I did it out of necessity, out of wanting to fix things that I thought were broken or could be streamlined. Occasionally, the resentment and bitterness from past events would creep to the surface, but I bottled it up and stuffed it back down. I had to focus on myself and getting to where I needed to be: employed in a meaningful career (with insurance). That was the endgame. Everything else seemed trivial, in a way.

*　　　*　　　*

Back in my college days, I was your average Type 1 Diabetic trying to find his place in the world. My diabetes was well managed and not an issue; it wasn't even a second thought. Now my livelihood was dependent on a diabetic alert dog. Boone was one of the main things that was keeping me moving forward and toward continuing my happiness. I had pushed past so much resentment and bitterness to get to this point to keep moving forward. Trivial took on a whole new meaning.

Around November, Boone was sick. He stopped eating and drinking. I took him to the vet and learned he had somehow swallowed a rock. A rock? In Arizona, yards and planters have rocks instead of grass or bark. Boone would need emergency surgery or risk bowel perforation. I got him set up for the procedure immediately, but I didn't have the money. I had to apply for a loan. My roommate, who had seen me at my worst, my best, and everything in-between, set up a GoFundMe page to help cover the cost of Boone's surgery. Moving back to Arizona came with significant changes. I had to find someone trustworthy to move in with because of my uncontrollable low blood sugars. While degrading, the arrangement became necessary for my survival. Thankfully, I had a friend who was willing to take on the responsibility to help look after me. It was such a kind gesture. I was very uncomfortable having my information out there for others to see and to be in need, but that was my reality. Within a few weeks, my roommate raised the entire cost of Boone's surgery. It was unbelievable that so many people were willing to help!

At this point, I really couldn't picture life without Boone. He had made such a tremendous difference in my day-to-day daily living that I grew accustomed to the pawing and his eyes begging me to drink my juice to save me from a diabetic coma. While Boone went into surgery, I spent a whole day without my trusty shadow by my side.

That same day, I returned to my kidney doctor for a follow-up appointment. It was that time of the year, and time for me to make my rounds with my physicians. I expected another bout of talking about low blood sugar with my endocrinologist and demanding answers from all my practitioners only to be met with disappointment and frustration.

I didn't have any pain and was pretty sure this doctor's appointment would be a quick follow-up to review my recent labs and images. I was sitting in the office when the doctor walked in and threw the lab and ultrasound reports on the exam table.

"Brandon! You're in kidney failure again," my doctor said. He knew to cut to the chase with me.

"Okay. Well, what do we do?"

"You need another surgery. Your kidney is the size of a cantaloupe and draining into what appears to be a lesion attached to the kidney. It's septic. And, we have to remove the whole kidney because it's dead. I'll make sure the same urologist performs the surgery that did it last time. He knows your body and is the best."

"Do we have to do it right now?" I asked him. My law school finals were approaching in a few weeks and if at all possible, I didn't want to take them late again or from a hospital bed. It was deja vu. *What on earth?* Except this time, I was also worried about Boone and his recovery. We couldn't both be down for the count. But, I trusted my kidney doctor to put my best interests first.

"We can wait until you complete your finals. We'll monitor you weekly and give you antibiotics to help control the sepsis," my doctor said. By now, he knew not to mess with my determination. If it could wait, he'd figure out a way to accommodate my schedule. I appreciated his understanding.

Thankfully, Boone's surgery went without any complications, and he bounced back to his dependable and happy self relatively quickly. I was three final exams away from graduation, and I couldn't believe my kidney was enlarged again. This should have been resolved last year with all the surgeries. I had the scars to prove it! It just didn't seem fair. Every time I tried to do something to better myself, my body decided to kick the crap out of me and throw another roadblock into the mix. The fickle nature of fate was nothing to dwell over. I would study for my finals, graduate, and take care of the surgery. It was just another thing on my to-do list at this point.

With no tubes coming out of my back this time, I completed my finals with the rest of my class. It was December 2016, and time to have my kidney removed. My mom and brother flew to Arizona for the surgery and to watch Boone while I was gone. While service dogs are allowed to go everywhere with their charges, hospital operating rooms are an exception to the rule.

By now, the routine of showering, getting in an awkward hospital gown, and being wheeled to the OR was all too familiar. It felt like a rerun of a really bad soap opera. Except in this rerun, you never knew what would happen. The beginning was always the same, but the ending could take a twist or a turn. I viewed surgery as a means to an end and that end was getting back to my life and all the wonderful things in it.

My surgeon attempted to remove my kidney laparoscopically, so the surgery would be minimally invasive. But the kidney was too large, the area was too delicate, and I had too much scar tissue from all the previous surgeries. Instead, they had to cut me open and fillet me like a fish with an 18-inch incision, much larger and wider than planned. They made the incision along my left side, removed the kidney and lesion, reattached everything, and stapled me back together. It was an extensive operation.

"Brandon, can you hear me?" the surgeon asked as my eyes fluttered open. I managed a tiny nod. Another surgery. Another hospital room. Another recovery. I hoped this would be my last.

"I couldn't believe what I saw," the surgeon said. "We took out part of what we thought was your kidney, but when we looked further there looked to be a whole other enlarged kidney there. *That* was your kidney. Basically, Brandon, your kidney created another kidney with stuff your body couldn't drain or reabsorb. Since the kidney and mass was so large, we had to cut you wider than expected to extract everything out. There was a lot of scar tissue to work through. You're going to be sore."

"Was it successful?" I asked my token question.

"Yes, but recovery may take longer than anticipated due to the amount of work we did on you, the risk of infection, and the size of the incision."

My body now had only one kidney, which would have to do all the work. I processed what the doctor had told me, my eyes wide open and my mind aware. The human body is an amazing thing. My kidney was so messed up it had generated an entirely new "kidney" type of thing, like building an addition on a house, to capture the fluid it couldn't maintain.

"Our hope is that your low blood sugars will decrease now that your body is not fighting the ill kidney and the lesion," the surgeon told me.

Oh man, I hoped he was right.

CHAPTER 9
Holiday Traditions

I was due to be done with classes and graduate early, in December instead of May, but I was healing and not feeling well. I had made it through the semester but didn't make it to the graduation. It is worth mentioning, my school wanted Boone and I in the front row with the staff and dean for the class picture, which I assume was a subliminal way to advertise the school as "all-inclusive." I saw right through that type of propaganda. A conversation about it would have been nice. Don't get me wrong, I appreciated the school accepting my service animal, but I did not like my diabetes to define me and didn't want Boone to be shown off. He was there for my survival, not as a novelty.

As for my future, I needed to figure out what was next. Law school was over, and I had to recover from this major surgery while studying for the bar exam in February. What if the surgery didn't fix the low blood sugars? What if I was disabled from chronic kidney issues and uncontrollable low blood sugars my whole life? How would I work? All of these things were out of my control and it was incredibly frustrating.

My mom and I spent four days in the hospital over Christmas as I continued to heal. My brother flew home the day after surgery. When I was finally allowed to go home, Boone started pawing at my legs. I was already having a low blood sugar episode. It was a major disappointment to find this out within hours of being released from the hospital. The next few days were immensely difficult. Boone continued to alert me, more often than ever. Every time I went to sit up, my body rocked with excruciating pain. I was supposed to be studying at least eight hours a day, five days a week, but I was in agony. Generally, I could push through things without a second thought. But my body just was not responding the way it always had before.

I'm going to take the rest of December off, allow my body to heal, and go full throttle in January, I thought. If I could focus my energy on healing this month, then maybe I could focus my mind on studying the next.

That was not the case. I kept having low blood sugars and passing out. I went to doctor appointments, and no one had any answers as to why my condition was deteriorating at such a rapid pace.

*　　*　　*

Healing from surgeries was not new to me, but I still didn't know what to fully expect. I went home for Christmas for a week before returning to my undergraduate school in Arizona. I had accepted the job as an RA again and wanted to help the new transfer students get settled in and feel like they had a place at the school. Also, I picked up a few shifts at the restaurant between Christmas and New Year's Eve. On December 31ˢᵗ, I finished up my shift at around 9 o'clock in the evening. I clocked out and walked to my car. As I sat down in the driver's seat, I flipped open my phone. There were 12 missed calls and every single one was from my mom.

My inner critic immediately wondered, *why didn't I bring my phone into work?*

I immediately called her back, but it went straight to her voicemail. I tried a few more times, but she didn't answer. Something was wrong; I just knew it. I punched in the number for our house line, but no one answered that either. *This is not good,* I thought.

My mind raced through possible scenarios. One scenario kept returning to the forefront of my mind and heart. It had to be my dad. Something happened to my dad—I felt it in my gut. A lump formed in my throat as one thought grew louder in my head: *My dad is dead.*

I went back to my dorm and kept trying to get a hold of my mom. I paced back and forth, the sounds of celebration and ringing in the new year in the background. Around 1:00 a.m., my mom finally called.

"Brandon, Dad was in a really bad accident. We don't know if he will live or die. They keep giving him blood. You need to fly here right away," she said within seconds of me saying hello.

I packed up a few things and headed to the airport. I had no idea what I'd be walking into. I sat on the plane in silence. How did this happen? What kind of accident? Is Mom okay? What about my brother and sister? The questions kept swirling chaotically in my head.

Once we touched down in California, my grandma Matilda picked me up and brought me home. My siblings needed things done at the house and the hospital's visiting hours were ending soon. As I walked through the front door, my brother and sister were calmly gathered in the living room. All we could do was wait. Wait for Mom to get home. Wait for morning to come so we could go to the hospital. Wait for answers. There was no use crying over the unknown. We stayed together, waiting.

When Mom arrived, I ran to greet her. She was pale, her eyes heavy and tired. It frightened me. I'd never seen her like that— she was the rock of our family. Whatever happened, it was deadly serious.

"We don't know much. Just Dad was in a really bad car accident. There are internal injuries, severe internal bleeding. He is in the ICU and the doctors are doing everything they can," she said. "We'll know more in the morning."

I tried to sleep, but it was a restless night. Early in the morning, we drove out to the hospital. There he was, lying in bed. Machines beeped rhythmically and a respirator was affixed to his face. Blood dripped into the IV lines hooked into his arms. He was completely black and blue and swollen. I barely recognized him. He looked...dead. My eyes drifted to the counter beside the window where his clothes, covered in blood, sat crumpled in a clear plastic bag.

What on earth had happened? How is he alive? I stepped out of the room, only to be surprised by a small crowd of people. They all seemed to be here for my dad. I glanced over my mom's shoulder and spotted three people I recognized. Standing in the far corner of the ICU visiting room were my grandparents and uncle. I hadn't seen them in years. These were the very people who contributed to our financial downfall and Dad's depression. Disbelief and anger overpowered my shock.

"Mom, what the FUCK are they doing here? They have no right to be here," I said, my voice raising. "They need to get the hell out and never contact you again!"

"We need all the support we can get. They got here last night," Mom said.

How did they make it to the hospital from Washington and Iowa before me? I was only a state away. I knew they were there because they felt guilty for all the horrible things they did to our family. There was no other explanation. Perhaps the only way they could free themselves of guilt was to come see my dad on his deathbed. Death would free them from responsibility. They don't deserve to be here, I thought. Where were they when Dad was suffering, in bed, and asking for help?

I glared at them from down the hall as they avoided eye contact. My mom stepped to block my view and reassured me that it was fine.

Before I could protest again, I felt my face. It was wet. I was crying without even realizing it. I wanted Dad to be at peace, but this felt like too much. I tried to understand what was going on in the situation, but was so shut off emotionally that I didn't know how to react. Then, it was like floodgates were opened and I started to sob. Just when I had finally composed myself, the doctors came in to check on my dad. I was eager for answers.

The medical team gave Dad 18 pints of blood in the first 24 hours. For comparison, the average adult maintains between 8 to 12 pints of blood at any given time. He needed an MRI, but was too fragile with the internal bleeding. Moving him was off limits. The medical staff had to address his internal and external bleeding first. He was in an induced coma, so they didn't yet know if he was paralyzed, and what was, if anything, broken. As it turns out, all the bones from his tail bone, through his right pelvis, and up to his neck were fractured or completely broken. The upper vertebrae of his neck were broken into pieces and jutted out of the front of his neck. It was touch and go. All we really knew was that they were trying to keep him alive.

We later learned he was driving his truck in the fast lane, heading back home from San Diego. He heard about an egg ranch around the area and thought it was a good idea to check it out. On the trip home, his truck tire caught the edge of the freeway, causing him to lose control of the vehicle, spinning and flipping over a couple of times. He wasn't wearing his seatbelt so as the truck flipped, he was ejected out the driver's side window. He flew 200 yards over and across the freeway, over four lanes of road, and landed in a seated position on top of a small tree. A branch punctured his rear end and shot up through his abdomen, piercing his abdominal wall before exiting out from his upper stomach. A good Samaritan, who happened to be an off duty EMT, saw what happened and ran to help before emergency personnel arrived. He tried to stop the bleeding as best as he could. He probably saved my dad's life at that moment. Thanks to him and the police report, we were able to understand the details of the accident.

As the ambulance took him to the hospital, the EMTs didn't think he was going to make it. He was losing too much blood and they couldn't figure out where it was coming from. Later, my dad said he remembered laying there repeating over and over in his head, "Just get me to the hospital, get me to the hospital. I am going to make it. I'm going to live."

The doctors kept Dad in the induced coma. Each day, they would reduce the anesthesia to see if Dad could pass a breathing and swallowing test. Then they'd return him to his coma. On the last day, something incredible happened. When they took him off the anesthesia he clawed at his respirator, trying to remove it from his face. Despite this being a good sign, the doctors restrained him and asked us to leave the room. When we returned to the room, my dad spoke for the first time, "I'm alive for a reason."

I looked at him closely and saw tears spilling from his eyes. My face flushed as tears welled up in my own eyes. He was going to fight. For the first time since his depression, from my perspective, Dad knew he was able to fight.

The accident signaled a turning point for him, both mentally, and physically. Finally, his blood started to clot and the bleeding subsided. The doctors removed his respirator permanently. All signs were pointing to progress except for the fact he did not pass the swallow test. All he wanted was an ice cold Diet Coke! He was only allowed ice chips due to having multiple surgeries lined up and his inability to pass the swallow test (which meant that liquids would be going into his lungs instead of down his throat).

The second thing he asked for was a pen and paper because it hurt too much to talk. It took a few tries but after gesturing as if he was writing, we were able to get him tools to communicate. The first thing he wrote was "WATER." We didn't know at the time, but he was on medication to suppress his salivary glands. His mouth was desiccated, and he longed for water but was not allowed to drink any. At one point he heard a toilet flushing and wrote "get me some of that water." He was desperate, but the only thing he could have was ice chips. No amount of water would have quenched his thirst at that moment.

"Everything looks stable, but we have to get an MRI completed to see what needs to be addressed first," one of his doctors told us. It was reassuring, but we wondered if they knew something they weren't telling us. With no clear answers, we wondered what to do. Was it okay to leave his side? What if he needed us? What if my grandparents show up again? What would Dad do?

My brother had just graduated high school. He came to the hospital several days a week with my mom. The nurses tried to feed my dad ice chips but once he could protest, he did. He wanted my mom or us kids to feed him. He didn't trust anyone else.

Grandma Matilda came by and spent time at the hospital and at our house. She helped take care of my siblings while Mom stayed by Dad's side. I proposed dropping out of school so I could be around to help handle things, but Mom was adamant that I finish school. The new semester had started, and it was only a matter of time before I'd fall behind. If she had said, "Yes Brandon, I need your help," I would have dropped out without a second thought; but she didn't. And so with Dad somewhat stabilized, my grandma pitching in, and my mom assuring me everything would work out, I returned to Arizona to face a new semester.

The whole ordeal made me begin to reevaluate my thinking and what I was striving for in life. Before Dad's accident, I just wanted to prove to everybody that whatever preconceived notions they had about my family and I were wrong. That's why I was always the responsible one. That's why I strived for straight A's in school. That's why I knew I could overcome anything thrown my way, that I could be successful without help. That's why I reached for perfection as much as humanly possible.

Dad had to wear a body brace and needed help with the simplest of tasks. There would be years of physical therapy in his future, but he was actually improving. Not just physically, either. The accident gave Dad a new outlook on life. He had a newfound will to live. This was opposite from the thoughts he had while depressed. Back then he wanted peace and to end the cycle of depression, hoping for death. Now, he just wanted to live and was willing to try. It wasn't an instant transition, but there were small signs demonstrating my dad was finally starting to face life past the veil of severe depression.

Something else happened during this time. All of a sudden people started contacting my family to ask about my dad and try to help us out after news of the accident got out. People who had previously shunned us and ignored our plight, the depression, and the poverty, suddenly found themselves shocked and appalled at our living conditions.

"I had no idea," many of them would say.

Like Mom said, we needed all the support we could get. But I found it ironic that during the ten years of absolute need, no one bothered to help when they knew the situation my family was in. I think it's because depression seems like something that should be handled alone. Depression is stigmatized as weakness and too often it is deemed to be the individual's fault. But a terrible car accident? That's just plain bad luck that people can relate to. The accident happened to my dad; unseen forces caused a tragedy, thus motivating people to step in and offer support.

I wanted to scream, "Where on earth were you the past ten years?" Instead, I kept my mouth shut and tried to stay grateful for the sake of my mom. When my dad got released from the hospital, he'd require around the clock home care. We wouldn't be able to afford a nurse, so Mom would have to do it all. If the community and friends and family wanted to make us hot meals and help with my siblings, I knew it would be better to be grateful than to question their motives.

*   *   *

During my recovery from surgery in Arizona, I didn't want the same people to know about my own health issues. I did not want all the attention that my dad received when he was hospitalized from fake well-wishers and a family I despised. Most of all, I didn't want anyone to know about my kidney surgery—except my immediate family. It made me vulnerable. Weak. I didn't like attention, especially from those that wronged me so much in the past. After witnessing the grand showing of "support" at the hospital for my Dad, I know I didn't want to give anyone a chance to suddenly decide to care. Managing this fake compassion, healing from my surgery, and studying for the bar exam would be too much to handle. I needed to move forward toward my goals, and for that to happen, I had to put myself into hyperdrive to get ready and pass the most important exam in my life.

CHAPTER 10

Clowning Around

Despite my best intentions, it proved impossible to properly study for the bar. I only got about one quarter of the study period completed. I did what I could. I counted down the days to the big test with an "it's okay if you fail, Brandon," attitude. It was a humbling mindset, but I knew something was still seriously wrong with my body.

My mindset of success, returning to D.C., making connections, and building a career slowly was being replaced with the goal of simply surviving each day. I started to care less and less about my plan of success because I couldn't tell what would happen in the next ten minutes.

I had never failed a test before, even in the direst of health circumstances, but I failed the bar. I vowed to retake it, but a small part of me was disappointed. I put every ounce of my being into meeting my goals. I tried and overcame every obstacle life and my body threw at me. I learned how to run a business starting at age 15. I learned how to manage living as a diabetic. I pushed up surgeries and pushed back surgeries. I hired an assistant for a day. I muddled through the fatigue in D.C., passed out at least twice (that I can remember) and even died just to name a few. But, I could tell I was getting worse. If anything, removing the kidney made things even harder because of the timing. I had spent the past two years dealing with abrupt low blood sugars and it was becoming more and more difficult to bounce back.

Still searching for answers, I saw multiple doctors. I tried to see physicians at the Mayo Clinic, knowing it was the best in the area, but they took only two specific types of insurance or cash. I had neither. I searched feverishly and made appointments with every doctor I could find, always taking the first available appointment.

Meanwhile, I needed a job to keep up with my living expenses. It was hard to find employment, since I was bar eligible instead of an official esquire, and I was expecting way too much of myself. Once I realized that and lowered my expectations, I found a job with a Phoenix law firm editing, researching, and writing memos. It wasn't the same level of excitement as my internship in D.C., but it paid and was still in the legal field. Each day I'd get up and drive to downtown Phoenix and complete an eight to ten-hour day before driving back home.

I worked overtime and, unfortunately, so did Boone. He was alerting me four to five times a day. It was interesting watching him work. He would be laying next to my bed, then start smelling the air, look at me and walk up to my bed and paw my arm. This was normal. It usually happened in the middle of the night. Boone would scratch the bed heavily to shake it and wake me up. I always had my stash of low blood sugar supplies, but I couldn't believe how often my sugar was dropping. It is a wonder Boone didn't show fatigue as well. Eventually, I couldn't even get up to drive to work. I just didn't have the physical or mental energy.

"I don't know what is going on with me and I don't feel like I'm doing a good job," I told my boss. I explained what was going on and asked, "What do you recommend?"

"Brandon, I think you're doing the best you can, but your health is the most important thing right now," she said.

I was a complete and utter failure. First, I failed the bar. Second, now I couldn't even complete simple research and editing tasks for my job. What good was I to anyone? Why was this still happening? I had so many surgeries in a short amount of time over something so small as a kidney stone. I had Boone. I was doing everything in my power to stay awake and alive, but nothing was working. What was I missing? I wasn't living. I was surviving.

*   *   *

After Dad's harrowing accident, I had decided to spend my time on myself. I needed to get outside of my head and have new experiences. I wanted to start to really LIVE. My continual failures felt like physical blows to my heart and soul. I had come through so much to get to this point.

I was required to complete a semester of student teaching for my credential after graduating from school in Arizona. I was assigned to teach twelfth grade government at a wealthy public school in the area. When you student teach, some master teacher's let you observe and slowly take over their role later in the semester. The master teacher I was assigned to had more than 30 years of experience. He had seen it all. Having a student teacher was a nice break for him.

"You'll be taking over the class from day one, Brandon," he said.

He gave me everything I needed and showed me how to prepare. I learned the roster, memorized the syllabus, got familiar with the schedule, and set time aside to plan each lesson.

On my first day, the master teacher introduced me to each period of my classes for the semester. The first time I took my place at the front of the room, I felt like something wasn't right. I scanned the eyes of my students and saw 40 desks full of young minds. My eyes darted across the classroom walls. There were no windows in the cramped room.

As I stood there, I got hit with a gut realization. If I had to do this for the next 30 years, I would be wasting my life. This is not for me. There has to be something different or more fulfilling. I hadn't even taught my first class yet, but in my heart, I just knew it wasn't what I wanted to invest my life into as a career. I didn't want to be stuck in a windowless room for the rest of my life. It wasn't physical labor. It wasn't like the egg ranch. On that first day, I felt like my skills were stifled, and I was already bored. Teaching was not experiencing life like I had hoped. I didn't want to be like that master teacher, decades into a career, eager for a slight reprieve from the monotony and bureaucracy of my day.

Even though I had already determined that I would not do this for the rest of my life, I still knew I needed to give my best to the situation at hand. I continued through the semester and tried to learn as much as I could. I implemented the same methods I did as an RA: I treated people with respect. I got to know my students and their likes and dislikes. I demonstrated an investment beyond just teaching the lectures. For some students, I learned I was one of the few people in their lives who consistently showed up every day. Helping them and giving back was rewarding. I even had students write me heartfelt letters on the last day of class saying how enjoyable my class was and how much it meant to them that they could count on me. I knew I was doing something right. Even the simple recognition I gave each student had an impact on their lives for the better. That hit me hard. I had faced a lot in this world already. My trials had led me to that point in time where I was a staple in the lives of my students. I was a dependable constant and it felt good to know I fulfilled that role in a meaningful way.

This sparked an internal battle. Teaching, I found, came naturally to me. Basically, you have to keep the students' attention for an hour through engagement, put on a performance, be larger than life, make the material relevant, teach, and encourage them to learn and ask questions or even research something they don't know. Essentially, I had to be a clown that could teach. But, the impact I could make was evident. I knew I could set my students up for success. I knew how to show up for others. My experience teaching inspired the question: "Am I living for myself or am I living for other people?" I still felt like I didn't want to teach forever. The pay was dismal, and I'd have to work multiple jobs just to afford basic expenses. It was a life of self-sacrifice that I wasn't sure I wanted to commit to in the long run.

Just to keep my options open, I began to explore other career opportunities. What did Brandon want to do? When I was growing up, I just wanted to run the egg ranch. I suppose that was still my goal in the long run, but for now I had to determine what could be next. A friend of mine said, "You should go to law school." I actually laughed at him. Me? Why? How? I hated school and I just thought there was no way—never, ever—that would be able to happen. I certainly wasn't smart enough, and I didn't even know anyone who was in the legal field. That crazy idea was probably the grandest goal I could ever set. I felt I would only fail, so why even try?

But, the law school idea stuck with me like an irresistible challenge. Could I really be a lawyer? Running all the scenarios in my head many, many times, I determined that I had nothing to lose if I didn't like law school. Plus, I could always fall back to teaching if it didn't work out. I was still trying to figure out my place in the world—some purpose that was missing. I had nothing to lose and I knew I'd prefer something challenging like law over restaurant management.

I decided to study for the entrance exam (LSAT), roll the dice, and see what happened. I somehow did well enough, not excellent or top notch, but well enough to submit a few applications. At least I could say I tried and wouldn't regret not trying later on.

I also took my certification course for my teaching credentials. I heard that the credentialing tests were very difficult. Yet, I passed. In fact, passing large and important tests was becoming a theme in my life, both literally and metaphorically. Now I was officially certified to teach ninth to twelfth grade social studies and could teach U.S. History, World History, Economics, and Government. I applied for a bunch of teaching jobs throughout the state. To my dismay, landing a job wasn't so easy. Due to the academic schedule I was on by student teaching, the semester after my graduation date, most school districts had already finished their hiring process months prior for the next school year. This was my mistake. No one told me the best time to apply for teaching jobs. Student teachers are often offered a position at the school where they teach. However, I was at a school district with no openings and would only have openings if someone retired. I secured a few interviews at charter schools, but to no avail. It was my fault to not ask more questions and ask how the hiring process worked. Then one day, my college called me with some great news.

"Brandon, we know a great school that you would be perfect for. You should interview," they told me. I thought, well, nothing has quite panned out yet, so I'll go for it. It was at a high school where I'd teach US History, World History, Government, and Economics. The interview went smoothly, and I was offered the job over the phone within an hour.

Once again, that little voice in the back of my head grew louder. Teaching is not for me. This is a mistake. What are you doing? DON'T DO IT! However, I needed the health insurance and the money, so I ignored the voice. Logically, this was the safest option at the time. I signed on for a year.

I was the entire social studies department. I was teaching all subjects, and had to create my own unique, informative, and engaging lesson plans, benchmarks, and exams. The school offered no help or support. I was an island left all on my own and "thrown to the wolves," as another teacher with years of experience mentioned. I was only directed to what I couldn't do, rather than what would benefit my students and I. By the final bell of the third day I wanted to quit and never return. Sure enough, it was the worst work experience of my life. The school differed dramatically from my student teaching school. I was taken advantage of and the school, and the students were a lot harder to connect with. Truthfully, this time, I wasn't set up for success which, in turn, meant it was even more difficult to set my students up for success.

Once again, I stuck it out for the remainder of the year while desperately seeking a way out of teaching. All I could think was, what had I gotten myself into?

To make matters worse, the school was a 45-minute commute to and from my house, due to rush hour traffic every morning and afternoon. I packed a lunch, but I had to help patrol the campus to prevent fights, tagging, drug use, and just "be seen" for the 30-minute break. I was miserable. I turned to food—a diabetic's WORST nightmare. Everyday I stopped to get fast food on my way home from work. Then I would later stop at a gas station to throw away the fast-food bag and drink cup, to hide the evidence from myself, my roommate, and anyone who would walk by and see the trash, before returning home. I knew I could do better. I was ashamed. However, having the time alone in my car and driving home was a good time to be in the quiet and unwind from the day. It felt good to have a belly full of comfort food.

Teaching so many separate subjects in one day with no preparation period was tough. Going into work on Sunday afternoons to use the copy machine and help prepare for the week was taking a toll on my health. That was a telltale sign I had a problem. But, it felt so nice and comforting to be full and be in the quiet of my car after a long and stressful day. My left eye would sometimes twitch if I didn't get to taste my fast food comfort. It dawned on me that I was using food to cope.

During Christmas break, I had almost an entire month off and didn't have to wear any of my work clothes. When I got ready after the new year to return to work, my favorite pair of black dress pants wouldn't button. What? Upon putting on other work clothes, I found most of my clothes felt tight and uncomfortable. My confidence in my appearance was slowly draining. That evening, after I found a baggy collared shirt to wear, I went to buy some new clothes that fit me. Ever since high school, I always had the same pant waist size. After trying on many pairs of dress pants, I asked an associate to measure my waist because there was something wrong with all the fit of the pants. She informed me that even though my waist measured at 37 inches, I would have to try a 38-inch waist size, since the dress pants weren't made in odd-numbered sizes. It made me feel frustrated at myself and not a little depressed.

I bought three new pairs of pants and five new dress shirts, so I didn't have to struggle with not fitting into my clothes anymore. I bought a scale, too. My first one ever. Once I arrived home, I put everything away then set the scale down in the bathroom. As I stepped on the white scale, the dial spun around quickly surpassing my normal 150-pound weight. It passed over the 200-pound mark and ended at 207 pounds. What? How? Why? This couldn't be right! This was way too heavy for my short stature and took away all my confidence. I was fat. This teaching job is draining my soul, I thought to myself, and the only way I can get any relief is through food. What was I going to do?

I realized I was hurting myself by resorting to unhealthy food for comfort. Doing so caused me to require more insulin. I decided the only option open to me was that I needed to find something else to do. I would need to find another job. I was angry at my college for saying the school I was teaching at would be "a great fit." I was mad at the school for working me to the bone. And most of all, I was mad at myself for going along with it, for letting it affect me, and for doing what I always did—pushing myself too hard to get the job done, no matter the toll it took on my health. It was time to make a change.

After the new year, I found out I got accepted into a few different law schools. I was very, very surprised. This new possibility gave me options to consider. Should I quit teaching altogether after this year and go to law school? Or, should I really make sure teaching is not for me? It was a risky gamble. Law school could be a horrible decision and then I'd regret leaving a stable job. Additionally, my health insurance at the time was excellent and required. I was able to afford my diabetic supplies with limited financial strain. I wasn't ready to give up that stability.

In the end, I weighed my options and decided the best thing for me would be to defer my law school acceptance for one year and give teaching another go. Thankfully, I got an offer to teach in a better, large public school that I quickly grew to enjoy. I taught 12th grade Government, just one subject. Best of all, my students needed to pass my class to graduate, so they were highly motivated to do well and cause the least trouble possible. For the first time since my student teaching experience, I really had fun teaching. I saw possibilities and thought maybe I had finally landed at the right place at the right time.

The school year went by in a fast-paced haze, and I was faced again with the decision to go to law school or continue teaching at this school I was comfortable at. I was happier. Was I completely fulfilled? No, but I felt this school was a supportive environment and the efforts put forth by administration matched my investment in the students. Most importantly, I had health insurance and was able to afford all my diabetic supplies. Even with insurance, I still had copays. Insulin is very expensive. Once you open a bottle or a pen, it has an expiration date of 30 days. Half my monthly income went toward doctor appointments and copays for medications. I didn't travel as much as I would have liked because I had to spend so much out of pocket. When I gained all the weight, I spent more money on food, which meant more money on insulin. I could get by on four bottles a month at $50 a bottle. With the weight gain I was up to six bottles a month. This influenced my decision greatly.

I deferred my law school acceptance once more and signed onto another year of teaching high school.

While I was in a much better space and was comfortable, I still found myself feeling unfulfilled. On top of that, my diabetic doctor told me that my cholesterol was rising and I needed to lose weight before things got out of control. I tried some diet plans but couldn't find one that I'd stick with. I met with the dietitian about what I needed to eat versus what I wanted to eat. My weight was getting embarrassing, and it was something that I didn't want to be concerned about anymore. Finally, I asked my doctor for advice. I was told to find whatever eating program I was most comfortable with, and stick with it for at least 21 days. He told me I'll know if I can stick with it or not after that.

I decided I was going to eat the high protein low carbohydrate meal plan that had been recommended many times before, with five to six small meals a day. I even set alarms on my phone. And, at the end of the 21-day mark, I was in the habit of eating small healthy meals five to six times a day. Within six months, I was back down to my normal weight of 150 pounds. I couldn't believe it. Now, my clothes were falling off of me, and I had to buy my old sizes again. I was proud of myself for doing something that was good for me. My blood sugars were much better and controlled, I was using half as much insulin, and I was gaining confidence in myself again. I had a job that wasn't sucking the life out of me, and I had the opportunities to do things for myself. I was living again, instead of just surviving and getting by.

But life was more than weight and work. I tried to get home to my family as much as possible. Usually, I made it back about twice a year and around the holidays. My brother was in college. My sister was working full-time. My dad was still slowly healing, though he experienced some mild memory loss and minor cognitive deficits. He finally got the green light to stop using his walker and cane. He even had a friend who stopped by the house to check on him after the accident, and later became a robust source of socialization. He drove Dad around and they'd talk about "the good old days," since they grew up playing basketball together. I consider that guy a sort of angel. With me in Arizona, Mom working at the restaurant, my brother at college, and my sister doing her own thing, my dad didn't have anyone to hang out with at the house or anything to look forward to each day besides slowly getting better. Thanks to his friend, he had something to do and someone to talk to during the day. I will always be thankful to my dad's friend for doing that.

About mid-way through my second year of teaching at the same school, I found myself yearning for a deeper sense of fulfillment again. Teaching just wasn't challenging enough for me. Not to mention, I was working part-time jobs on the side, including as a front desk clerk at a hotel three nights a week and some construction jobs here and there so I could afford all my bills and have extra spending money to have fun. As a teacher you get holidays and summers off. Once I lost weight, I went with a group of friends to Mexico during one of my summer breaks. I didn't go very many places during the school year; I'd rather save up for a big summer trip. Although insurance kept me teaching, I felt there had to be more to life.

I briefly considered going back to school for something different or even getting a job at a restaurant where I could work my way up to manager before looking over my law school acceptances again. One of the local schools was now considered a top tier law school. I was shocked I even got in. It was a very competitive program. It's crazy how the person who grew up on an egg ranch and said he'd never go to college, graduated, became a teacher, and was now entertaining the idea of law school.

I still didn't know who I was or what I wanted in life. Really, I was just going through the motions again. I was surviving, not thriving, like I promised myself I would do after Dad's accident. The fundamental values that made me the person I was at the time, just rolled over from one massive responsibility to the next. I was always the kid stepping up, doing everything by the book, helping out where I could, shouldering the responsibility that was really meant for other people much older than me. I had lived a complete life in just a few decades. Each adventure had traces of the experiences that came before it. Running the egg ranch at 15 and working as a teaching assistant and a teacher all primed me for leadership and management skills at a young age. I had to keep records, organize things, make sure people were doing what they were supposed to be doing, and compile reports, among many other tasks. My work always came with immense responsibility and required something ingrained in me since I started walking: dependability.

But, that didn't answer who I was at my core. It merely demonstrated the things I could do, not the person I could be. I knew it was time for a change. I had to shake up my life if I was ever going to find my way and my place in the world. I made up my mind to go big or go home.

My LSAT scores were set to expire, and at the conclusion of my second year of teaching I had to decide once and for all if I was going to law school or not. I pulled up my law school acceptance form on one computer screen and my teaching renewal contract on another computer screen beside it. I looked at the two documents, two different paths leading to different destinies.

My eyes darted back and forth between the screens. Finally, I took a deep breath, grasped the mouse, and clicked on one of them.

I accepted my enrollment into law school.

Without a second thought, I turned off the computers and felt at peace with my decision. Hell, I even felt excited for the first time in a long time. A new adventure and experience was awaiting me. Maybe I'd hate it and be way worse off, but I was prepared to lose everything to gain something. I had no idea where that path would lead, but I knew it was a change I needed.

Health insurance was a huge factor in my decision. In March 2010, the Affordable Care Act (ACA) changed my life. Every job that I had done in my life, from the egg ranch to teaching, every decision I made, was based on health insurance. I chose teaching and working at the Olive Garden for the insurance to cover my diabetic supplies and appointments. With the ACA in place, I could no longer be denied coverage because of my preexisting condition. In a way, it was the first time I felt the government working for me. I knew people who were fundraising just to buy bottles of insulin because getting health insurance was too expensive. This was life changing for me and so many others. The ACA didn't solve all the problems, but it did open new doors. Now, I was free to make decisions based on other values. I had no idea what I was doing, but I called the number to sign up for insurance based on my income as a full-time student. Much to my surprise, it was a simple process and I began receiving affordable health coverage. Things were now much easier to navigate, and it provided me the opportunity to continue furthering my education.

*   *   *

Gone were the days when access to health insurance was my greatest burden. Now it was trying to figure out what was happening with my body and diabetes. My new job would be tackling a gauntlet of doctor appointments. I had a calendar with everything meticulously set up and my list of questions and responses were permanently etched in my mind. The questions were for the doctors. The responses were for me, since every doctor asked me the same damn thing. Ever the self-advocate, I hoped I could find an answer to my low blood sugar issue. Summer catapulted into fall and I had seen eight different endocrinologists, four different kidney doctors, a natural holistic doctor, Eastern religious healers, and more. Nothing helped. It was always the same. No one understood what was going on, and I was having a hard time correctly expressing that there was something wrong with me.

November rolled around and open enrollment for health insurance began. I was low income and on Medicaid. Insurance was expensive to pay cash at full face value, so I had to take what I could get. I made the mistake of not applying for different insurance or even properly shopping around for an income-driven plan. Instead, I kept the health insurance I had and planned a visit to see my parents in California.

One of the things I knew when I returned from D.C. to Arizona was that I had to live with someone who would be willing to check on me to see if my blood sugar was low or not. I had Boone, but I needed more. I moved in with a friend who understood she would basically need to make sure I was alive each day.

It was a typical Thursday morning, except I wasn't up early like I usually was. Years of getting up early for school had my internal alarm clock programmed for 6:00 a.m. By 8:00 a.m., I had not emerged from my room. My friend knocked on the door and found me lying in bed, unresponsive. She called 911.

The next thing I knew, someone was yelling, "He's breathing!"

What the hell? I thought, *Am I dreaming?*

The fog started to lift as I looked around. I was in my bed, in my room, but surrounded by strangers and my friend. The strangers wore uniforms. They were EMTs.

"Sir, we couldn't find a heartbeat and you weren't breathing when we arrived," one of them told me. "Your roommate said you're diabetic and we gave you multiple glucagon kits."

"Oh," was all I could say.

"I have never seen anything like this in my life. We were going to stop working on you. You were a goner. I swear you were out for at least ten minutes. Can you hear me?"

"Yeah," I replied.

I was the miracle for the day. I have no idea how or why I survived. I couldn't believe this happened to me again. Twice my body had shut down on me, and twice it had started back up. I thanked my roommate for her quick response. Had I lived alone, I would have been a "goner." This near-death experience shit was getting out of hand.

When I went to bed that night, I felt nervous. I wasn't sure if I'd wake up, so I tossed and turned through the night thinking of everything that had gone awry. It wasn't so much the fear of dying as much as it was the inability to know how to solve my life-or-death problem. No doctors had come through for me yet, and, despite tons of research, I couldn't figure out what to do next.

CHAPTER 11
A Brittle Answer

A short time after coding on my roommate, I made a planned visit to see my parents in California around the holidays. Dad was doing well, working at a golf course, and moving around as best as he could. My brother was married, and my sister was living her best life. My mom was in the middle of painting the interior of the house. Wanting to feel useful, I offered to help, just like I used to help around the ranch. Boone stayed close as I climbed up and down the ladder and painted as much as I could. Little did I know, manual labor would take a huge toll on my body. That evening, I went to my room and curled up in a ball. My body felt like it was weighed down by cinder blocks. My eyelids were glued shut and my head pounded.

With my legs tucked close in a fetal position and Boone a few feet away, I succumbed to the exhaustion and fell asleep. This is what would happen if I did anything physical. My body was unable to recover. It was like I was in a constant state of low blood sugar. I spent two whole days in bed.

"We have to figure out what is wrong with you. You look like you're withering away," my mom said.

"You don't look good," my dad agreed.

I felt awful as I saw their worried expressions. I never wanted them to have to worry about me, but here we were. Having a bit of my energy restored, with all my effort, I could finally sit up. Even Boone stared at me with his concerned brown eyes. I realized my mom and dad had no idea how bad I really was until they saw me in that condition. They didn't know about the Metro incident, or the presentation, or the cruise, or any of it.

"This has been going on since my D.C. internship," I confessed. "The doctors keep telling me to eat a graham cracker before bed and watch my insulin."

Sparing them the most frightening details, I told the story of the code blue on the cruise, my long "nap" on the Metro, and my most recent brush with death in my own home.

"Why didn't you tell us sooner?" my mom asked, her voice cracking slightly.

"I didn't want to worry you," I said, admitting failure in that department as well. I didn't want to peel back the layers of my own vulnerability. I didn't want to show weakness when I had been such a strong person my whole life. Admitting I was weak was so embarrassing, albeit humbling.

"It's our job to take care of you," my mom said softly. My parents were not mad. They knew deep down that even if I had told them sooner, nothing could be done. I was a medical mystery of the worst kind.

Gradually, I got out of bed and started to plan my next move. I had no money. My parents had no money. My rent was $350 a month. It was just a room, but in a house with someone who agreed to help look after me. I also needed money for food, gas for the car to drive to my doctor's appointments, Boone, and medication. I wasn't sure what to do. I was between the proverbial rock and a hard place. There had to be another option. I was not ready to simply give up or give in to the disease that was destroying me from the inside out.

"Maybe I should move back home," I said to my mom and dad. "That way, someone can always keep an eye on me."

My parents looked at each other, pausing thoughtfully for a moment. "As much as we'd love that, all of your doctors and medical records are in Arizona. It would be best to go back to them instead of starting from ground zero," my mom said. Dad agreed. They knew my roommate was there, and I had Boone to help as much as possible.

They were right. It would be a pain to have all my records transferred to California. Not only that, but scheduling new appointments with specialists and having to wait for months to get in to see them would only hurt me. Time wasn't in my favor. But, how would I afford to live? I was waiting for my disability to be approved and trying to come up with some way I could bring in additional income that didn't involve a lot of physical movement or travel. I was disabled, broke, and had a wonderful diabetic alert dog to feed as well as myself.

I laid back down on my side and stared out the window overlooking the patio. The red padding on the chairs seemed so cheery. *Why had I never noticed that before?* Boone rested his head on the bed. He knew I was feeling bad. There had to be more doctors in Arizona to try. I shamefully applied for disability, and hoped I would be able to afford to live again. Even in my thirties, it seemed like poverty was chasing me down. I didn't need much, but the basics were still expensive. Asking for my parents' advice, having them in my most vulnerable state, and needing help, put me in a tough spot. I didn't ask for help. I always figured things out. This time, however, the mental and physical exhaustion made it too hard to fight back on my own. It felt like I was starting over.

I tried looking at it another way. I was given a second chance at life. I should have died multiple times from Diabetes already, but I didn't. I am still kicking. Why? I decided to work toward not caring so much what other people thought about me, especially my family. Instead, I would try to discover what I thought about myself first and continue seeking out medical experts until I had an answer.

Success was always my number one goal in life. But, what I failed to realize was that I would do whatever it took for me to be successful. I wasn't afraid to chase after my dreams. However, I could be mean and even an outright asshole, if I felt people were wrong about something or if they tried to impede my ability to get to where I wanted to go. Now, I was with a dog that saved my life on a regular basis. I was alive. I had a few people who really cared about me, people who helped me out of kindness. I didn't care about success in that way anymore. Success now meant that I woke up in the morning.

After my epiphany, I made my way to the living room. It felt good to move, though it took much of my energy away. My mom must have heard me because she called my name from down the hall, and I turned around and walked to my parents' bedroom. *Guess I'm a kid all over again,* I thought.

"I have an idea," she told me triumphantly.

"Alright," I told her, genuinely curious.

"Your grandma Matilda is going to lend you money to continue your appointments, pay your rent, and feed yourself and Boone," she said. "I told her what I've witnessed these past few days and what you shared with Dad and I. You can pay her back when you get better."

I didn't know what to say. I hated that I needed the help so badly. It was degrading that I'd have to accept this "handout" and eventually be on government disability. I didn't consider myself disabled, but I absolutely was. I also had no other options in terms of income. My grandma was—again—coming through for me at the best possible time.

"She offered without hesitation," my mom added, sensing my apprehension.

My grandma Matilda knew that if my mom was asking her for money, then it had to be something very serious. I was always my grandma's go-to person if she had something that needed to be fixed or if she wanted to know something. I was someone she trusted. I was so thankful for her generosity and kindness. For me, she lived and acted in the manner that I expected, and tried to live, as family should. Without her help, I wasn't sure what I would have done.

A few days later, when I was well enough to travel, Boone and I flew back to Arizona. I found a new endocrinologist who was willing to try everything rather than writing me off and telling me to eat more. She agreed something was seriously wrong with me. Our first treatment option was to see if I could keep my blood sugar as high as possible. Sometimes, the doctor explained, the endocrine system will reset itself if there are no low blood sugars for at least two months. Plus, I had antibodies working against the insulin, which added to the issue. It was the first time I had heard of insulin antibodies, but it was not the last. She certainly presented a new idea, and I was desperate to try anything—even though it was an underhanded way of saying "eat more."

At first, I could keep my blood sugar high in the 250s (which isn't very high, but high enough to not worry about being low). Yet every single time, I would crash dramatically and Boone, the ever watchful, perfectly trained, life-saving dog, would paw my leg. My doctor suggested my body wasn't processing food correctly. "It's probably gastroparesis, a common Type 1 issue," she said. She sent me to a specialist to determine if that was the culprit. I had to consume a hard boiled radioactive egg while a machine monitored my digestion. She was disappointed when she called to inform me that I did not have the condition. She was right about my body not processing food correctly, but it was emptying correctly. Once again, it was a dead end, inspiring more questions than answers.

Finally, in January 2018, I was given a new diagnosis. "Brandon, you're a Brittle Diabetic," she told me. "A Brittle Diabetic is someone who has hard-to-control diabetes and is characterized by wide variations of blood glucose levels." *No shit,* I thought to myself.

Keeping my blood sugar at high levels with no lows wasn't working. Every day, I'd still have low blood sugar. How is this going to work if I am supposed to keep my blood sugar high, but it won't stay high even when I eat as much as I want?

I tried a different doctor. The office was small and could have used a face lift or a genuine renovation. The staff called me back into the exam room and I awaited the new doctor. Fortunately, my test results, labs, and medical history followed me wherever I went in Arizona.

"Brandon, I have all of your records here. I've gone through everything, and I've seen your condition before," the doctor said.

For the first time, in a long time, I felt a glimmer of hope. Was she about to tell me something I had not heard before? *Please don't tell me to eat a graham cracker,* I thought.

"You need a pancreas transplant. If you don't get one, you will not live beyond two years."

Wow, straight to the point. I blinked. Before I could open my mouth to speak, she continued.

"There is nothing you can do when you're in this state. It can't be undone. You've been dealing with this for over two years and it can't go on for much longer. Your body will simply stop recovering because your brain shuts down due to lack of sugar in your blood. This can only happen so many times before it doesn't restart. The low blood sugars are also destroying the connections in your brain. If we were to do an MRI, it would show grey matter. You're doing everything you can, but you need a transplant. And soon."

"Thank you," I said in earnest. Finally, an answer to the two-year long medical mystery also known as my life.

"Do what you have to. Beg, borrow, steal, whatever it takes. I've even had patients who went to other countries and paid cash. One low blood sugar is deadly. I don't want to scare you, but this is a very fragile situation."

She referred me to Banner Transplant Hospital, the only hospital in Arizona that accepted Medicaid, and sent them my records. I was interviewed by phone for them to determine my eligibility for an evaluation. Instead of a courtesy call, I received a curt letter in the mail informing me I had been denied because I only had one kidney and wouldn't be able to afford the surgery because it was not covered by insurance.

My heart sank, I was devastated. They wouldn't even allow me to see a doctor and learn more about the transplant options. They made a judgment call that I couldn't come up with the money and the institution did not want to work with such a "high risk" patient. I didn't understand why a pancreas transplant wasn't covered by insurance. It was medically necessary and qualified under all definitions. After doing research, I found out that the Affordable Care Act put pancreas-only transplants under the optional coverage of transplants. That meant insurance companies, Medicaid, and Medicare were not obligated to cover them.

If I needed another kidney and a pancreas, it would be covered. Or if I needed a liver and pancreas, it would be covered. I just needed the pancreas and for some reason that was "special" and ineligible. Finally, I knew what I needed. I just had no idea how I could ever get it. I started researching the cost of going to another country.

CHAPTER 12
Change of Heart

"Here's the deal," I said into the phone to my parents on the other side of the line. "Banner rejected me as a candidate. The only other transplant hospital in the state is Mayo Clinic. They are top notch for transplants, and known throughout the world as being one of the best medical centers, but they only take two types of insurance or cash."

"We will figure this out," my mom said.

"The other option is going to another country, like India, and paying cash. It's the fastest way to have it done, but the success rates and quality of care are questionable," I continued.

My dad yelled, "You're not going to have a transplant in another country if you can have it done at Mayo!"

That was easier said than done. The kicker was if I had signed up for different insurance back in December, and paid full price in cash instead of having Medicaid based on my lack of income, I would have had the proper plan to cover a pancreas-only transplant, or so I thought. Now it was too late to change my coverage. I quickly considered moving to any other state so I could qualify to change my insurance position, but the pancreas-only coverage was only available in Arizona. Go figure that I was in the only state with the insurance coverage I needed, but couldn't get access to it.

I reached out to my sister-in-law's aunt, who was a top dog health insurance lobbyist working to help change denial claims into acceptance claims in D.C. She contacted everyone she knew, including the insurance company CEO and governor, but came up empty. Banner could legally reject me and the Affordable Care Act could legally deny me coverage for a life-saving surgery. I appealed everything and received a letter from my insurance's CEO office. The letter explained that even though the insurance company stated it covered anything medically necessary, and my pancreas-only transplant was medically necessary for my survival, they would not cover the consultation or procedure or medications related to a pancreas-only transplant because it was an exception within the Affordable Care Act.

Straight to the point, a pancreas transplant can only be covered by insurance if it can be added onto another covered transplant. Pancreas-only transplants are rare and one of the few exceptions to "medically necessary." Just my luck. As a diabetic, there are plenty of "interventions," including monitors and medications, to manage the disease. I was an extreme case, a rare case. The pancreas-only transplant has a high rate of rejection. A pancreas/kidney transplant is preferable because it increases the odds that both organs will not be rejected.

Blow after blow, I was getting more discouraged. How is it that the health system set in this country to save lives could be the very system that failed me and mine? The cost of the transplant would be astronomical. It was mind-blowing that insurance wouldn't cover any part of it. I always had trouble getting things covered with insurance, like insulin and test strips, so I was used to dealing with denials and appeals. But, for some reason, this particular denial was one I couldn't shake off. I had to keep living, but not in the low blood sugar mind fog. Life didn't take me on this crazy roller coaster only to have me fade away into nothingness now. I had to keep searching for answers.

Dismayed, I returned to my kidney doctor for my regularly scheduled follow-up appointment.

I relayed my diagnosis and he nodded confidently. As I sat in the office, my doctor took out his cell phone. "Let me see," he said, punching in a number. I watched quietly, not exactly sure what he was up to.

"Yeah, that's what I thought. He's been a patient of mine for years," he said to the person on the other line. "Brittle diabetic. Yes. One kidney. Great, I'll tell him."

I looked up expectedly.

"You're going to the Mayo Clinic. I know three people who had the same problem as you. They all had the pancreas-only transplant and today they are living normal lives. One of my colleagues is a transplant surgeon at Mayo, and I'm referring you for a consultation. Having one kidney is not an issue and doesn't disqualify you from getting a transplant. I don't have a say in the decision of your transplant candidacy, but I will be sure to send my medical clearance along with the referral over to Mayo for you. This is a fast pass to the first part of the process. Do whatever it takes to get the pancreas, Brandon. The patients and friends I've seen who have a pancreas transplant are thriving."

"Really, just like that?" I said, relieved to be catching a break for once.

"Yes, I've done all I can do. Now the rest is in Mayo's hands," he said confidently.

Before leaving the room, he mentioned that he met me two years earlier, and he couldn't believe the difference he saw in my complexion and demeanor.

"I can tell you are on your last leg. You won't be around much longer if you don't have this transplant as soon as possible," he told me solemnly.

To me, it seemed like a transplant was a no-brainer. However, no one else, besides these two doctors, really understood.

In March 2018, I had a ticket into the Mayo Clinic because my trusted kidney doctor referred me. My endocrinologist, who knew I needed a transplant, couldn't get me an appointment with Mayo because she didn't have any connections. It was my kidney doctor who came through for me once again.

I was still relying on the generosity of my grandma to help me with my day-to-day expenditures. Barely surviving financially and physically, I felt I had to keep fighting. I was unable to do anything productive, so getting healthy and having the transplant was the only way to change that. Having applied for disability months ago, and denied three times, I had no choice but to hire an attorney. To my delight, this attorney happened to be someone I went to law school with. I had no idea until I walked into her office. Ever the professional, she worked on disability claims and got mine in the emergency hearing line. Even with an emergency hearing request, I'd have to wait until after the new year for a hearing. Another system originally built to help me was doing quite the opposite.

Time is such a precious resource and I wasn't sure how much of it I had left. Wasting no time whatsoever, I made my appointment with Mayo for the initial consultation. Just to make the appointment, I had to pay $780! It was crazy. It cost $780 just to see if I could be considered for a pancreas-only transplant. With few options at my disposal, I called my mom. Between the money my grandma gave me, some money my mom had from her job, and a credit card I had, I was able to pay for the appointment. I prayed this much needed money was not thrown at something that would fail me too.

With the appointment requested, the people at Mayo said they'd let me know if the appointment was confirmed. Two days later, I was permitted to go through the consultation process. The patient advocate carefully explained what the impending weeks would look like. I'd undergo stress tests for my heart, an X-ray, CT scans, MRIs, you name it. This was all to make sure I was healthy and viable to receive a transplant. I asked multiple times if having one kidney would hinder my chances. On every occasion, I was told it would not be an automatic disqualification. With extreme caution, I got my hopes up, but there was still one major issue: nothing would be covered by insurance. If I were to proceed with the consultation, I'd have to come up with additional funds. So they directed me to call Mayo Clinic's financial services department.

"Hello, thank you for calling Mayo Clinic. This is Shawna, how can I help you?" a kind voice asked.

"Hi, my name is Brandon Mouw. I'm about to undergo a consultation to determine if I'm a candidate for a pancreas-only transplant. I'd be considered uninsured because I don't have the insurance Mayo Clinic accepts. How do I make it all work out financially?"

"Sure, I can assist you with that, but I'll need more information," Shawna said.

We reviewed the logistics: my birth date, diagnosis, what place of the consultation process I was currently in, my financial status, and more.

"Thank you, Brandon. So, as you may know, pancreas-only transplants are quite rare. Generally, patients receive a kidney and a pancreas at the same time. It's fortunate but unfortunate. If you needed a kidney as well, then the transplant of both the kidney and pancreas would be covered with your current insurance here at Mayo. Currently, there is one insurance company that is covering the pancreas-only transplant that we accept, but you won't be able to sign up for the plan until open enrollment in December. You can always give the insurance company a call and to inquire about paying full price for the plan. It wouldn't hurt to check all options. However, based on your records, you need to be listed for the transplant ASAP. Also, your physicians are all in agreement that you only need a pancreatic transplant," she said.

I listened intently, holding my breath.

"The pancreas-only transplant waiting list is very short. We have three people currently listed. In general, the waiting list is three months to three years, but most people receive their transplant sooner than expected. I've witnessed people who are called in the day after they're listed."

"Okay, so how do I get listed without insurance?" I asked her.

"It will be $20,000 for the consultation and that includes all tests, labs, and follow-up diagnostic procedures. You will have to pay that upfront to have the full consultation scheduled."

I let out a tiny whoosh of air, hoping Shawna did not hear it.

"Alright," I managed.

"Once that is complete, your consultation results will go in front of the transplant committee. They will determine if you are a candidate for the surgery. In the event you are approved for transplantation, you will be put on the transplant list based on your blood type, which is called UNOS, then will have to pre-pay $250,000 for the surgery."

Whoosh. I let out the remainder of the breath I had been holding.

"Wow, okay. That makes sense," I said. After all, I realized it wasn't going to be cheap. I just had no idea it would cost the price of a small house. "Thank you for your honesty."

I liked Shawna right off the bat. She provided me with the facts and was honest about what to expect and how much it would cost. She didn't sugarcoat it. She didn't beat around the bush. She didn't give me a list of scenarios. She told me exactly what I'd need to do to live. If I didn't have the transplant by January, then I just might be able to purchase insurance from the marketplace to cover it. However, I still needed $20,000 to proceed with the full consultation to see if I could even be a candidate for the surgery.

At that moment, dying wasn't my worst nightmare. I had no fear of death and no fear of failure. Instead, an uneasiness crept up inside of me. It wasn't the fear of an impossible task...it was the fear of asking for help. There was absolutely no way I could do this alone. I was going to have to ask for help. In fact, I was going to have to ask people for money. It went against every single thing I had spent my life fighting against. I worked tirelessly to be self-sufficient and independent. But at that moment, I had two choices: succumb to vulnerability or succumb to death.

"What do you recommend to raise these funds?" I asked Shawna. I'm sure she had gotten this question many times before.

"Some people ask their family members and friends. I've seen a few patients successfully raise some funds through on-line fundraisers like GoFundMe. There are also personal unsecured loans through banks which could be an option."

Could I get a loan? I had a ton of student loans and very limited income. My credit was okay, but I wasn't sure I'd be approved for such a substantial loan. The whole thought of reaching out to others to ask for help made my skin crawl.

Immediately after getting off the phone with Shawna, I called the Arizona insurance company to see if I could enroll in the plan that Mayo accepted and that covered pancreas-only transplants. They told me about all the great things the insurance plan had to offer, only to point out that I was ineligible to sign up for a new insurance plan because it was not open enrollment and I did not have a qualifying event. (A qualifying event is losing health coverage or moving to another state, to name a few.) I'd have to wait until the end of the year to enroll, and the coverages would likely change by then. There was no use messing around with insurance right now. So, I called my parents and gave them the facts, just as they were presented to me.

"Other than grandma, I don't have anyone else I can ask," my mom said. My dad was quiet.

"I could call my friends, I guess," I said reluctantly. I had several family members who had plenty of money, but I had not seen or talked to them in over 20 years. There were family members who still owed my dad money from his "investments" long ago, but I did not even want to consider them as a viable option. Why would they help now?

The next day my mom called me back. She had a little bit of news.

"I talked to my friend about your situation," she said. "After hearing the whole story she suggested you write a letter explaining exactly what is going on. You make sure you highlight the seriousness of the situation. No one knows what you're going through, or what you need, or that you're dying. No one."

I felt my whole body tense up. This was not the news I was expecting. I kept things private for a reason.

"People think you're a successful attorney. You keep everything private to a fault," my mom said in a matter of fact way. "Write the letter, send it to the family and a few friends of the family to start. What do you have to lose?"

My dignity. My pride. The walls I had built around myself and my heart all these years. My sanity. I could name a few things.

"I will not do that, and why are you telling people about this?" I asked firmly, but with confidence rather than anger. I could hear her sigh at my stubbornness.

"What choice do you have, Brandon?"

"I despise these people to my core. I don't want to tell them about all my problems and that I need money. They never helped us before. What makes you think they will help us now?" I asked her.

"Think about it," she said.

I did. It went against everything I believed in, but with no other option, I decided to write the letter.

I'm Still Kickin'

To whom it may concern:

I am writing this letter to you out of pure humility because I have run out of options, and time is of the essence. Since June 2015, when I had two kidney stones removed and was septic, I have been in a downward spiral regarding my health. This letter explains what I am going through, what my options are, and asks you for help.

BACKGROUND AND HISTORY

Ever since I was diagnosed with Juvenile Type I Diabetes at age three, I have always been able to be a well-controlled diabetic with no complications. Low and high blood sugars were a regular and ongoing thing, but they were correctable and manageable. In January 2016, after my seventh surgery to remove scar tissue from my kidney and to reconnect it, I began having extreme low blood sugars. During this time, I was taking law school classes in Washington, D.C., interning at the Capitol, and not realizing what exactly was going on with my blood sugars—I just began not feeling well and noticing that I was having more lows than normal. During the Summer of 2016, I stayed in Washington, D.C. to be a legal intern at the Department of State. While I was there, I began to start missing/forgetting hours of days, passing out (one day got on the train after work to head home, and woke up six hours later all because of a low blood sugar), and really started to see a difference in what was going on with my blood sugars, but not knowing what was going on.

I wrote about the incident during my presentation in front of colleagues and how I got Boone (and the ways he has saved my life). I detailed how my blood sugar monitor was 30 minutes behind live-time due to the blood capillaries attached to the skin receiving blood last. Due to this, low blood sugars came on within minutes with no warning, hence Boone.

In December 2016, I was in kidney failure and septic again, and had a lesion growing off the kidney because it couldn't drain. I was taken to surgery and had my kidney removed, which was supposed to solve all my blood sugar issues. However, it only solved the kidney issue—not my blood sugar issues.

I graduated law school in May 2017, and began working at a law firm in Phoenix. However, it became evident that I was having issues remembering important things, being able to wake up when my blood sugar was low, and, again, going unconscious and losing track of time at work. Therefore, I had to stop working, and began to focus on finding out what was going on with my health.

NEW FINDINGS

Since January 2017, I have continually had more and more low blood sugars. I do not recognize or feel the low blood sugars happening because they happen suddenly, without explanation, and without pattern. Each time my blood sugar goes below 70, my brain starts to shut down non-essential functions. So, I lose my ability to think clearly, logically, or normally. Moreover, the longer the blood sugar stays low, my brain shuts down other non-essential functions in order to reserve the energy for my heart and lungs. Every day, my blood sugar goes to 40 or below. The issue is that my body can only restart so many times before it can no longer recover from so many restarts.

I shared the struggle of going from doctor to doctor with no answers. I talked about the insulin antibodies and my diagnosis as a brittle diabetic.

Since having hypoglycemia unawareness, I have died and been resuscitated twice. The first time happened while on a cruise with friends where I was found unresponsive while getting a massage, not breathing, and had no heartbeat. It took the emergency services over eight minutes to resuscitate me with the defibrillator. The second time, a few months later, was when my roommate checked on me because I wasn't up in the morning. I would not wake up and wasn't breathing. She had to call 911, and I had to be resuscitated again. The low blood sugars are not a joke. The diabetic doctor says that it is the riskiest illness to deal with because one low blood sugar will cause death, whereas high blood sugars take years to cause death. Unfortunately, I have low, low, low deadly blood sugars every single day.

I live with the fear of going to bed each night and not waking up. Because I am at the mercy of what my body does, there is no consistency or trends or preventative treatment. Every low blood sugar is random, and hits me hard. To understand what an extreme low blood sugar does, imagine yourself at your absolute sickest, not being able to think, walk, and talk, while being dizzy, and in a state of absolute confusion. That is what a low blood sugar feels like. It takes me hours to recover from low blood sugar. I cannot think clearly, answer the phone, or do anything productive. All I am able to do is lay in bed and wait for my brain to start functioning again.

At this point, I have gone through every type of treatment to help prevent the low blood sugars from happening, but all have been unsuccessful. Due to all the low blood sugars, I may have long-term brain damage because parts of my brain that get shut down everyday cannot recover. In turn, the amount of gray matter in my brain is continually growing and will never be able to be reused. Furthermore, I am continually low in sodium because of the hypoglycemia and autoimmune issues, so my body doesn't break down essential elements, which means that I am at extreme risk for seizures. In addition, my one good kidney is starting to leak protein, which is due to the stress of the low blood sugars on it.

Right now, the only form of treatment—and my only hope—is to get a pancreas transplant. The pancreas transplant will, if my body does not reject it, solve all the issues I have. However, my insurance will not cover the procedure, and I cannot pay cash for the surgery. So, I require help.

OPTIONS

Here is where I am at with these issues: I must have a pancreas transplant to live. I went to another appointment with the diabetic doctor on May 16th, and she said that I have to get the transplant by any means necessary—beg, borrow, or steal. She said to find insurance that covers pancreas-only transplants, pay cash, or go to another country where it's less money. The doctor doesn't know how much more damage my body can take before it cannot recover, less than two years, and if I wait until I can switch insurance it might be too late. They said that I can borrow the money, and pay everyone back when I am recovered because I'll be back to normal and fully functional.

Like any good lawyer, I put all the evidence on the table, chronicled my options, and extrapolated the insurance issue in great detail. I highlighted the fact that paying $250,000 plus the $20,000 cash was my absolute BEST option for survival. I also offered the possibility of paying for a pancreas transplant in a different country (something I researched heavily).

> *As of right now, those are my options to receive the pancreas transplant to live. Having the cash is my best option, since time is of the essence. Or, at least having $20,000 to pay for the consultation, tests, and to get on the transplant list will put me leaps and bounds ahead of where I am now.*
>
> *I would prefer to have the surgery done at Mayo Clinic, but am more than willing to go to India because of the price and expeditious process. However, I truly do not believe I will survive eight months for open enrollment to begin the process of getting on the transplant waiting list; then, another three months to three years for the transplant. My best option for survival is to get on the transplant list right away by being able to pay in cash.*

CONCLUSION

> *I did not ask for this to happen to me, I did not do this to myself, and I have always taken care of myself. I do not drink, smoke, or use drugs. This is just something that happens after 30 years of having a chronic disease; and I am extremely embarrassed that I do not have insurance that covers this procedure and have to ask for help.*

The impact of what I have been dealing with, with brittle diabetes, has been unbelievable. Never did I think I would be in this place of not being able to help myself. I am desperate for help of any kind. Therefore, after going through all the options and knowing I cannot wait for a long time, I am asking for financial help to get this transplant done as soon as possible, as my life is literally on the line. Once I am up and running and healed, I will use my law degree to get another well paying job and pay everything back.

Please contact me as soon as possible to go over the options, as time is of the essence and I need your financial help to live.

Thank you for your consideration,
Brandon Mouw

I felt sick to my stomach. I reread the letter, feeling worse with each word as the crippling weight of vulnerability washed over me. I had now put all my weaknesses on paper for the family to see. I was exposed. Everything was exposed. I wanted to live, and I had to do what was necessary.

Using certified mail so I'd know when the letters were delivered, I sent the letters to about eight family members and friends of family. My mom told me to let her know if I heard anything back. I asked her to do the same. A few days later, my dad called asking if I received a response yet. The answer was no, but I knew everyone received them. After hanging up with him, my phone rang. It was a number I didn't recognize but the area code looked familiar.

"Hello, this is Brandon," I said.

"Oh yeah, Brandon. Tell me what is going on. I got your letter," my grandpa said. It was my dad's dad, and we had not talked in years. I bit my tongue. I wanted to say, "Did you read the letter, it explains everything?" Instead, I rehashed exactly what I wrote.

"If a few people could give me a few thousand dollars each, I'd be able to see if I'm a candidate for the transplant," I said.

"Okay. Well, that's not good to hear. You know, I can't help every grandkid out of their messes. You better stop asking me for anything because I'm not giving you any fucking money," he shouted over the phone before hanging up on me.

What?

Every terrible thought I ever had about myself and everybody I ever came to know rushed over me. It was suffocating. My greatest fear came true. It was what I expected. But still, I was shocked. I was embarrassed. I needed to get away and start all over and have everything done the way it was supposed to be. This was the very reason why I didn't want to ask for help. What had I gotten myself into?

In the meantime, my loyal roommate, who put together the GoFundMe page after Boone's surgery, decided to start another fundraiser for my transplant. I was leery about having my "needs" out there for everyone to see, but I was grasping at straws to see what could or couldn't happen. No one had donated yet, but at least it was another possible avenue. In the wake of my grandpa's rejection, I felt like anything involving family was a waste of effort. Those people had never been there before. Why was I expecting them to be there for me now? My grandpa sure had a way of making a person feel like less than dirt. With all the means in the world that was built upon the backs of his children, he could not be bothered. I know it's not my place to judge, but I was not in a good head space. To this day, I wish I was proud to be his grandson. I expected the remaining letter recipients to either ignore me or call to say something similar. Still, I was determined for this transplant to happen. I had a desire to keep trying. I was not ready to give up. I was alive for a reason. There was no room to let doubt take hold.

The next day my dad called. "We got a check in the mail," he said. "It's for $20,000." "You're kidding! From who?" I asked.

"Someone you would never expect," my dad said. I could hear him crying through the phone.

This person must remain anonymous, but I can say I had not seen them in many years. I couldn't believe it. They came through for me. It disproved everything I felt and thought about my own vulnerability. I had a place to start, a foothold, in getting some answers about the possibility of a transplant and my survival... finally.

My dad told me he'd overnight the check so I'd have it in the morning. When I hung up with him, I called Mayo to let them know.

"I have $20,000. How do you want it? When can I get an appointment?" I asked happily.

"We can start scheduling you for next week," they said. "And we take cash, credit, wire transfer, and cashier's check."

I went to my bank with the check and cashed it right away. I walked out with a manila envelope full of cash and drove straight to Mayo Clinic. It was surreal. I prayed nothing would happen to me on my way to the clinic. I walked into the financial office and greeted Shawna with a huge sigh of relief.

"I have never seen someone do this so quickly," Shawna said as I set down the answer to all of my problems on her desk.

She smiled. "I already called the scheduler. Told them this is an ASAP situation. Expect a call soon."

"I'm ready," I said.

CHAPTER 13
Medical Mayhem

With adrenaline and optimism coursing through my veins, I left Mayo Clinic filled with the sense of knowing that I was doing exactly what I was supposed to be doing. It seemed impossible, but somehow, it was happening. It was the first time, in a long time, I felt such profound and deep emotion. The reality and realization of what I had been provided with, was so real that it was like jumping into an ice-cold swimming pool. I was shocked by the generosity of someone I had once written off as selfish and too good for my family and I. This person genuinely cared about my well being. Under normal circumstances, I don't think I would have given them a second chance at being back in my life; yet I reached out in true need, and they showed up for me.

There aren't enough words to fully encapsulate my gratitude for the anonymous person who donated the $20,000.

I'm Still Kickin'

What did I do to deserve such a gift? Now, I had to pass a gauntlet of tests, labs, and diagnostics.

True to her word, Shawna put a rush order in for my fully paid consultation series. The next day, the scheduler called and asked when I'd like to start. I told her I'd take the first available appointment. Time was of the essence. She booked an appointment for me with a kidney and pancreas doctor who manages patients like me. My medical history would be inspected with scrutiny, and even though they had all my medical records, I'd be answering many of the same questions repeatedly. But I didn't mind. I would do whatever it took for a new pancreas.

I saw the kidney doctor, as well as a patient coordinator. I checked in with my financial coordinator, Shawna, then met with a dietitian. We discussed my current diet and any necessary dietary changes if I had the surgery. It seemed unbelievable at first, but apparently I'd be able to eat just about anything if the surgery was successful. I wouldn't need Gatorade or Mentos, and I could eat what I pleased, like a healthy 33-year old non-diabetic.

Next, I met with one of the Mayo transplant surgeons. She was soft spoken with a thick Minnesotan accent. Within seconds of meeting me, she fell in love with Boone, who laid obediently underneath my feet. One of the first things she told me was that someone had just been called in for a pancreas-only transplant, and they were getting prepared for surgery upstairs. She also mentioned that the waiting list is very short. *That's too good to be true*, I kept thinking.

"Can I even be a candidate with one kidney?" I had asked many people before, but I had been denied so many times in my life, I wanted to be sure.

"Of course. Why not? Your kidney appears to be functioning just fine," she said in the softest, most kind voice. "Especially if you have the pancreas transplant, then your kidney won't be under the stress of diabetes and chronic low blood sugars, and will stop leaking protein. However, the post-transplant medication you have to be on for the rest of your life is hard on the kidneys. If your kidney failed and you went on dialysis, do you have anyone in your immediate family who would be willing to donate a kidney to you?"

"Yes, I do. In fact, I've had people who have offered to donate their pancreas," I said.

She laughed, a soft chuckle that made me smile just listening to it.

"I feel you are a candidate for this surgery. I will be recommending you for surgery to the committee," she stated confidently. "Now, it's important to know that you may get called in for a transplant, and arrive for surgery, and be all ready to go, only to find out that something is not right. Usually, it has to do with the donated organ. But, we will inform you about what is happening as we are aware. When that happens, you will go back home and wait for another call when there is a match. People usually get called in three times before the perfect match is found."

They could call me in as many times as they needed to; I didn't care. I felt my eyes burn as tears started to form. Just hearing her words brought me peace, even though my body and life was in absolute chaos. I held back my tears and took a deep breath. I felt so seen and so understood in that moment. The people at Mayo Clinic knew what I needed. No B.S. Everyone so far had treated my condition as the serious and life-threatening issue that it was. No one had told me to eat a graham cracker or gave me false hope. I was exactly where I was supposed to be.

Elated, I made my way to my last appointment of the day. It was with a social worker coordinator who would evaluate my ability to sustain a transplant. *This should be easy.* I had spent my entire life properly managing my diabetes until it couldn't be managed anymore. I ate right, took excellent care of myself, worked hard, and always tried to reach my personal goals. I loved my family and would do anything for them.

I recently asked for help in a huge way and I had a network of friends and my roommate who served as a solid support system. Out of all of my consultations, I felt confident that this one would be the quickest.

"Brandon, how do you handle your medication?" she questioned in a tone typically reserved for small, petulant children.

Immediately I knew this evaluation would not be like the others.

"I take my medication regularly as prescribed and have always been a self-sufficient and independent diabetic until my brittle diabetes took over," I replied calmly.

"I see, and how do you handle stress?"

"Well, I take deep breaths or go for a walk. I've dealt with some very stressful situations over my lifetime, from a young age, and I tend to just handle it, focus on what I can control, and work on my stress from that angle."

She scribbled a few notes down and then flipped the page in her chart. She let out a low "ohhh."

"So, I understand your insurance does not cover this procedure," she said flatly.

"That's correct," I affirmed. "But, if I'm a candidate, I will have the means to pay for it."

"Do you have the cash on hand?" she asked, with a hint of skepticism in her tone.

"No. To my understanding, I am finding out if I can be a candidate for a transplant. If I am a candidate, and know how much the procedure will cost, I will have the funds available at that time," I answered. This conversation seemed to be taking a dark turn. I didn't have the money nor knew how I would get it, but one way or the other, I was determined to make this transplant happen.

"So, you're not going to be able to afford the medication to care for an organ that someone's deceased loved one gave to you?" she asked sharply. "You do realize this is considered a gift and you're obligated to care for it as if it is your own!"

That was a pretty intense accusation directed at someone going through one of the most challenging things of his entire life. I could literally go to bed, have a low blood sugar, and not wake up despite Boone pawing me relentlessly. It would all be over. Here I was at an award-winning medical facility with people who could literally decide if my life was worth saving or not, and this coordinator was challenging me as if I didn't understand what was at stake!

"I did not say that. Just because I do not have the funds for the surgery at this moment does not mean I don't have the cash to purchase the medication afterwards. I don't even know what is expected, and that's why I'm here. I've taken care of myself throughout my entire life. I always had the ability to afford the expensive insulin, insurance, and test strips and diabetic appointments. I'm not sure why this cash issue is such a problem at this very moment," I told her.

"Everyone says that. The truth of the matter is that cash patients are the riskiest because they simply don't have the cash up front. Very few do or can prove they have it. They are all talking," she lashed back.

This woman did not like to be challenged. I'm not sure what other patients did in my situation. Did they give up on the *transplant*? Did they call a loan shark right there in the office? I would never know. What I did know was that this woman was getting very angry with me for no good reason at all.

"Where is your caretaker?" she asked, abruptly switching topics.

"In California, why?" I replied.

"They have to be here," she said.

"Oh, where does it say that on the paperwork sent to me? I know my caretaker must be present during surgery, but I believe it is optional to have them with me during the consultation process," I told her.

"It's on the website. It is recommended your caretaker attend all your appointments. Your caretaker is not here today," she said, almost triumphantly.

Lady, I have a different understanding of words since I graduated law school. Mandatory and recommended do not mean the same thing. And, if you are going to throw words and jargon at me, you, the professional, better be ready to defend the words used.

"Mandatory or recommended?" I asked her.

"It states recommended," she lowered her voice in defeat.

"I see, well to be honest, since it was not mandatory, I didn't think it was necessary for my mom to fly out from California for these appointments," I offered. "I don't even know what the outcome will be, and I already paid the $20,000 for the consultation process in cash."

"I see how it is. You don't follow instructions," she sneered, writing something else in my chart.

"Okay, well, I am just here trying to see what is possible and if I am a candidate. Had I known how important it was to have my caretaker present, she would be here. This is a non-issue. Would you like me to call her? You can speak to her over the phone, or she can fly out and be here first thing in the morning. Also, my roommate can be here in 30 minutes if I call her. I am demonstrating that I can make the necessary things happen," I offered, annoyed by her interrogation.

"No, it's fine. Let's go over the cost of your prescription medications and discuss how you will afford them."

For the next 15 minutes, we went back and forth. She informed me that a post-surgery medication cost $7,400 or something ridiculous for a 30-day supply. I have an app on my phone that is used to get the best price available for my medication. I looked up the same drug and discovered it would be $220 for a 30-day supply. When I showed it to her, she scoffed.

"That's impossible," she almost yelled.

"I use this app all the time and have been using it for years. If you're unaware, it demonstrates how out of touch you are about how things work in this world. I've navigated the healthcare system since my diagnosis at age 3." I had enough. She was relentless and we were getting nowhere.

"Fine. What is your highest level of education?" she asked, pivoting to another topic once again. I was getting whiplash from the abruptness of each turn the conversation took.

"Juris Doctorate."

"Doctorate?" she asked, once again doubting me. "Okay, does anyone in your immediate family have cancer?"

"No."

We went through some family history questions before she slammed the chart down on her desk. She pivoted her body toward me and said, "I don't think you're ready for this surgery. I'm not recommending you for the transplant at this time. You need to see a psychiatrist because I don't think you can emotionally handle the responsibility of this transplant."

I was pissed, shocked. I felt personally attacked, and was refused the opportunity to be heard or to even have a polite conversation. This was not how it was supposed to be. This treatment, let alone from a social worker, was abhorrent. I wanted to yell or scream or walk out of the room and find a witness to see the nonsense that was occurring. But I knew I couldn't. You can't reason with someone who has it out for you simply because other cash patients couldn't care for themselves. And, did every cash patient fail to receive a transplant? I'm not everyone else. But, there was no way that this woman was going to deny me my life saving surgery. It would be detrimental if I was told one kidney disqualified me. But me not being "emotionally competent" was total bullshit. This was not something for a social worker to decide. I had to get ahead of the damage I knew was coming.

"What's your supervisor's name?"

Her mouth popped open, and her face flushed red. I stood up to gather my things. On my way out of the room, I snatched a business card off the table. I had a very important phone call to make. But first, I dialed the one person I trusted at Mayo the most—the financial coordinator.

"I just had a great day. I was in a great mood. Then, I met with someone who is extremely unqualified to determine what is going on. I was attacked because it was assumed I wouldn't be able to pay for my medication. Under what guise have I proven that to be true?"

"I've never heard of anyone having an experience like that," Shawna said.

After briefly venting, I left a message with the social worker's supervisor. They called me back in a few hours.

"I'm sorry to hear you had a negative experience. I've never had a patient complain. The social worker's notes paint a very different picture than what you're saying. We will definitely assign you to a new coordinator. Unfortunately, in this situation, it's too late...."

"...Too late for what?" I asked, panic rising in my chest.

"She has already pushed your paperwork onto the next phase. She has recommended you see a licensed psychiatrist before continuing your transplant evaluation."

"Everyone has been phenomenal here. I've been treated with respect and kindness. But this one person has made my otherwise perfect experience absolutely miserable. She is supposed to be helping me understand the transplant process and my ability to cope with it, but all she did was argue and refuse to listen to me or have a reasonable conversation. I think this would fall under the medical category of refusal of care, especially because her opinion is not based on my medical history. She is basing it on her experience with other people. Due to this incompetence, I do not want her opinion to be the criteria holding me back from being a candidate for this transplant. I also want to petition that her opinions be stricken from my file and she not be allowed on the committee that decides if I can be a candidate or not."

"Of course. Well, she is on the committee, and there is nothing I can do. I think you should follow her recommendations to show you can follow directions. Here is the information for the psychiatrist. Go see them and then we'll get you back on track."

I sighed. I didn't have a choice. True to my nature, I booked an appointment with the recommended psychiatrist for the first available slot. Before I could be seen, however, I had to come up with another $890 for the appointment because it was a non-routine appointment that the $20,000 didn't cover. *Testing me much?* Luckily, I had just received a very small tax refund from working at the law firm the previous year.

The psychiatrist was nice. We discussed many different elements about my life, as well as my mental and physical well being. We talked about what went on in my last appointment with the coordinator. I remained calm and controlled as I rehashed the initial consult and pleaded my case as to why I was a responsible, independent, and perfectly capable individual.

"We'll give you a call soon," she said dismissively.

I left and called my parents to update them on the progress. The next few days went by without incident. Boone, of course, alerted me to my low blood sugars as I kept my phone glued to my side, waiting for my next direction. The transplant committee met every Tuesday to discuss the qualifications of transplant candidates. That afternoon, I received a call.

"Brandon, we absolutely believe you are a candidate for a pancreas-only transplant," the head coordinator said.

"That's great when can I –"

"But," she cut me off, "your psychiatrist recommends you have three months of cognitive behavioral therapy."

"I'm sorry, what?" my heart sank.

"It says here the psychiatrist is concerned that you have issues with being confronted," she said.

"Did the psychiatrist relay the whole story? Did she write down that I was attacked for standing up for myself when I was being berated by an unqualified employee who provided a terrible experience at Mayo? I'm told I have a very short amount of time to live. In that amount of time, every single setback takes away from my quality of life and chance for survival," I explained.

"We're aware of your situation, Brandon. We took that into consideration, but the committee's decision stands. You're technically listed, just as inactive. Get three months of therapy (12 sessions total, one session each week), fax in the records with the therapist, and make an appointment with the psychiatrist in three months. You have to do a total of three months of once-a-week Cognitive Behavioral Therapy. When you have accomplished that, then we will put you up for reevaluation."

Shit.

Out of all the potential roadblocks to the transplant, this was not one I considered a possibility. I had no choice but to find a therapist and pray I didn't die during those three months. All because the social worker didn't like to be challenged and, as I later found out, the psychiatrist she referred me to was a friend of hers. At this time, I realized I should have just played dumb and not stood up for myself because I most likely would have ended up actively listed. However, I did stand up for myself, like I always have. This time, it may have cost me my life.

I found a qualified therapist through my insurance. She was a former attorney who retired and went back to school to become a therapist. After I explained to her the whole ordeal, she asked if we should sue. We laughed. As much as I wanted to, I knew the transplant was far more important. We met weekly and checked the boxes. Cognitive behavioral therapy is really just replacing a negative thought with a positive thought. For someone who spent his whole life never scared of surgery or death, I was a champion at such thinking.

On top of this new roadblock, I had to be treated for latent tuberculosis, something I may have been exposed to as a teacher, but never manifested. Ironically, it required a three-month treatment—exactly the number of months I had to be in therapy.

I felt like I had the weight of the world on my shoulders. A few days after I found out I'd have to be in therapy for three months, Mayo called to inform me I was physically approved for transplant; all my tests had been passed without issue and I was a perfect candidate for transplant. *Go figure.* They also told me instead of paying $250,000 as a lump sum, I could pay $100,000 up front and then later prove I had $150,000 in a trust. That would confirm my surgery once a viable pancreas became available.

It seemed impossible, but I wasn't going to go down without a fight. Then, something crazy happened. About one week after I posted that I was approved for the transplant, but needed to raise the funds to pay for it, my grandma (the wife of my grandpa who told me off) called my dad. She asked him how much money I needed. My dad told it to her straight, "He needs $250,000 total and if he can provide $100,000 upfront, they'll move his application along."

"Okay, get me the wire number. I'll send over $100,000 to Mayo Clinic tomorrow," my grandma told my dad.

"You're saving his life!" my dad replied, genuinely surprised by her generosity. We weren't sure what caused her change of heart. It may be due to me being the first male grandson born in the family. Or perhaps she wanted to do something meaningful. Whatever the reason, I was in shock and awe. Another completely unexpected gift.

When my dad told me the news, I immediately called Shawna.

"I have $100,000 ready to be wired, what do I do?" I told her excitedly.

"Brandon, how did you make this happen?" she asked.

"I didn't. Other people are making this happen. If people are offering, we're going to take it," I said, knowing I needed all the help I could get. She gave me the wire number and instructions, and I texted it to my grandma. Part of me wondered if it was too good to be true. After my grandpa's brush-off, I didn't expect anything from that side of the family. Would he put a stop to his wife's good intentions?

I didn't have to wait long to find out. Shawna called me the next day and confirmed receipt of payment. When I completed my therapy in three months, I'd be good to go. It was the definition of a miracle. I'd just have to survive for the next three months.

I learned that people need to know your weaknesses when you ask for help. People cannot help you if they don't know what is going on. You have to trust that not all people are bad and let them in. My friend who was setting up a GoFundMe page on my behalf asked to use a shorter version of the letter I sent my family and friends. She said if people knew I was close to receiving the transplant, they would be willing to donate out of urgency. So, in a matter of weeks, I went from no one in my extended family or friends knowing what I was going through, to the entire world having all the intimate details.

After my friend published the GoFundMe page on Facebook, donations started trickling in. I'd get $25 here and $300 there. I started receiving larger donations from people I didn't even know. I'd get $25,000, $15,000 then $10,000 sent directly to the trust. Many donations came from people I never even met. They saw my information on someone's Facebook page that they shared about me. A second cousin sent $25,000 without saying anything to me. As the donations poured in, the entirety of emotion I had muted throughout my life started breaking through the surface. I was moved beyond belief by everyone's generosity. I questioned it. Why would people want to take their hard-earned money and help me? Who was I to these people? What had I done to deserve this generosity? If that original donation of $20,000 never came to fruition, I don't think the ball would have started rolling. None of this would have been possible. It took the generosity of one to inspire others. One thing was for sure; my perspective on life was dramatically changing.

I spent the next few months diligently attending my therapy appointments. We went through Cognitive Behavioral Therapy workbooks, and then talked. We discussed my low blood sugar, how being a diabetic from the age of three impacted my life, how being closed off from the world for such a long time then opening up changed what I thought about life, and how to enjoy my life right now in the present. We talked about my plans for after surgery and what I wanted to do with my life once all of this was over—when I wasn't sick and on the brink of death anymore. My therapist made an unbearable experience go by quickly and smoothly.

With my mental state "in check," my physical state continued to decline. On most days, I was going out of it. My roommate would find me wandering around the house, talking nonsense, and being confused about simple things. Boone was constantly pawing me and alerting me to my low blood sugar. I was in complete survival mode.

By October, I had my last therapy appointment. Through word of mouth and keeping people updated on my progress, and social media, I raised $105,000 through GoFundMe. My grandma had wired the $100,000 to Mayo Clinic. It was enough to move the process along as I worked to raise the last remaining amount. I had proven my financial stability to Mayo and completed the required therapy. My application went before the transplant committee once more. I was worried I would have to do all the physical tests and examinations over again due to my continual low blood sugars and the toll it took on my body, but thankfully, that wasn't the case.

"You are now actively listed," the coordinator told me. I was so relieved. I couldn't believe I did it. I had made it so far and so many people were willing to help me. People helped me not only financially, but also through kind words, thoughts, and prayers. All of it! The most unexpected people came through for me. Despite years of people avoiding our family in our most dire time of need, humanity and kindness still existed. There were still people in this world who had a heart. I wasn't drifting through life alone anymore. Many people proved that they were present all along, even when I wrote everyone off and trusted no one. I felt undeserving of the kindness but it gave me a new purpose for living. There were so many times I could have given up, but I didn't. I fought like hell. I felt like I moved mountains. There must be some reason I was still alive, and it looked like I might get to discover why.

CHAPTER 14

A Christmas Miracle

I was told it could take between three months and three years before I might get the pancreas transplant. Since I was actively listed, I had to go to my doctor to complete blood tests every 30 days. When you are put on the UNOS transplant list, you are registered based on your human leukocyte antigen (HLA) and blood type. When a donor becomes available based on blood type, the transplant team mixes your blood with the blood of the donor to see if the blood does anything suspicious. Sometimes the blood can reject the donor blood, an early indicator of organ rejection.

I dutifully submitted my samples in October and November. Then came December...my not so magical month. I had my blood drawn for Mayo as usual, but December has long had a history of surgical procedures and health issues for me. I was waiting patiently for the call that could change my life forever, even knowing that it could take up to three years. Since I was actively listed, I wasn't permitted to be more than two hours away from Mayo Clinic. Well, I could be; it's just that if I was further than two hours and there was a match and I received a call, then I'd be too far away for the transplant at that time. It was not a risk worth taking. At this point, it didn't matter. I was out of it too often, my body was failing, I felt like crap, and I didn't have the mental or physical energy to do much. Needless to say, my family understood why I couldn't travel home for Christmas.

I had some friends play the waiting game with me. Knowing I couldn't spend the holidays with family, they devised a plan.

"Brandon, let's go up north to the mountains and snow the day after Christmas. There is a little town we can stay in and we can get away, get some fresh air, and have some fun," my friends offered.

My roommate offered to watch Boone. I wouldn't require him to be with me since I would be with two trusted friends who would keep an eye on me and knew what to do when my sugar was low. It was exactly two hours away. I wouldn't have to fly or drive. Plus, constantly monitoring my phone and feeling my heart skip a beat every time it rang or vibrated was exhausting. I really did need a break.

"Let's do it," I said. *Things can't get any worse.*

The three of us piled into a car on December 26th and headed north for two days. It was bitter cold but it felt nice being out of my room. We walked around the quaint downtown, bundled in layers. The snow was supposed to start around 10:00 p.m., so we had made it to town just in time. After we walked for a bit, we found a small bar and tucked ourselves inside. Warmth, food, and friendly company filled our evening. Constantly being reminded to eat carbohydrates and sip on my Gatorade allowed time for me to play darts and pool. Then a chill settled upon the bar and I started to get cold.

"Hey, let's go somewhere else or go back to the room to put on another layer," I said.

"Another layer sounds great."

They knew I shouldn't be alone. The last thing we needed was for me to pass out on the sidewalk. We gathered our things and headed back outside and to our room. Quickly, we put on another layer and agreed that we were going to another bar and restaurant that we passed on our way back to the apartment where we were going to stay. As we crossed the street and walked into our new destination, I realized I had drunk all the Gatorade I had on me. I had to go back to the car and grab a few more bottles. As one friend went in to find a place to hang out in the bar, my other friend accompanied me to the car parked a few blocks over. I hadn't taken more than four steps when my phone began to ring. I pulled it out of my coat pocket.

A 480 number. That's Mayo's area code.

"Hello, this is Brandon."

"Hi, is this Brandon Mouw?" the caller asked.

"Yes, it is."

"Can you confirm your date of birth?"

"Yes," I said, and confirmed my birthday.

"Are you ready for a new pancreas? We have an identical match. How soon can you get here for surgery?" they said excitedly.

Holy shit. Is this really happening? What are the odds...

"I'm exactly two hours away," I said, nervous this would disqualify me. A perfect match sounded too good to be true. Did my jaunt to the north cost me this life saving organ?

"Okay, well, hmmm, let me check with the transplant team and I will call you right back," the lady stated.

I hung up and turned to face my friend. "I got the call!" I explained that I had to wait for a call back since I was two hours away from Mayo. We quickly walked back to the bar as I popped a few Mentos into my mouth.

"Let's go back to the apartment just in case," I told them. I wanted to be warm and relatively quiet with good reception for this next call.

Five minutes later the 480 number called back.

"This is Brandon," I said confidently. I held my breath. My heart pounded rapidly in my chest. I felt my face flush with warmth. I almost felt like I was sweating even though I was cold.

"Good news. Two hours is perfect timing. The surgeons are en route with the organ. Get on the road and give me a call back when you have service. We're going to do a pre-surgical application over the phone, so you'll be ready upon arrival," she told me.

"I will be there as soon as I can. Talk to you soon. Thank you so very much!" I turned to look at my friends. "Guys, this is it! I might be getting a pancreas! I'm going to get an Uber and head back down right now."

"Brandon, no. We're going to drive you," my friend demanded.

"But we're out here on a break and having fun. You don't have to stop on account of me. An Uber will be fine," I assured them.

"Hell no. Let's pack up. We're going together."

We threw our belongings back into our backpacks and bags. Within what had to be less than four minutes, we were on the highway heading south. Once we got to an area with more reliable service outside of the mountains, I called the coordinator back. It was pitch black, around 7:30 p.m. and about to snow, but my friend drove as quickly and as safely as possible.

"Okay Brandon, and when was the last time you took this medication?" the coordinator asked me. She had tons of questions including when my last low blood sugar was and what I had to eat most recently. Finally, she asked, "Who is your insurance provider?"

"I prepaid in cash," I told her. By now I had raised all $250,000 with the help of my grandma, friends, family, strangers, and of course the GoFundMe page.

"It's not coming up that you prepaid in cash..." she sounded concerned.

"Call the financial coordinator, if you don't see that I prepaid. She said that it's noted on my charts and if there was ever a question that she would be the person to contact."

"Okay, she is gone for the holiday, but I'll give her a call."

Literally two minutes later, my phone rang again.

"Brandon, I spoke with Shawna. You're confirmed and good to go. Please meet us at the ER entrance. Tell the front check-in desk that you're Brandon Mouw and you're here for a transplant. Everyone will know what to do."

"Got it, what should I bring? Is this a sure thing? Should I make sure my caretaker arrives as well?" I asked.

"Just come as you are, and, yes, your caretaker is required to be there when your surgery is complete. However, it's never a guaranteed thing."

Thankfully, I had been through enough surgeries and knew what I should bring. Whenever I'd go in for a major procedure, I always had my cell phone, wallet, and a change of clothes. I called my mom. She was out to dinner with her friends.

"I got the call!" I told her as she stepped away from the dinner table to a quieter location.

"I'm not sure if I'm actually going to have the surgery. I was told that this could happen at least three times before I actually go under the knife. But, Mayo says my caretaker needs to be there when I get out of surgery and right now all signs point to go. They said it's a perfect match."

"Brandon, that is fantastic," she said. I could hear the surprise in her voice. We hung up so we could use our phones to research flights. There ended up being one flight coming out of the Ontario airport. It was leaving in less than an hour. My mom abandoned her dinner, rushed home, and headed straight to the airport. She actually had to pay for her ticket right at the desk and walked directly onto the flight.

My friends dropped me off at the Mayo Clinic Emergency Department entrance. I jumped out of the car, put some things in a bag from the trunk, and walked inside.

"How can I help you?" the triage nurse asked.

"I'm Brandon Mouw and I am here for a transplant," I said slowly, loudly, and clearly. I could see my name written largely on a piece of paper behind the glass at the desk.

"Great, go stand right there, Brandon," she said pointing at a spot on the wall as she picked up the phone.

A few seconds later, a nurse opened the two large doors leading into the hospital and called my name.

"Hi, let's get you back and ready for surgery," she said excitedly.

"Is everything a match?" I asked.

"The blood type and HLA were matches. That's as close as you can get," she said as we walked into a large surgery prep room.

Suddenly, my room filled with people. A nurse assistant came in to remove my clothes and put me in a gown. An assistant surgeon came in, reviewed my vitals, and began explaining the procedure to me. Another nurse gently held my arm as she inserted an IV. On my other side, a nurse drew blood for a final test.

"So, we're going to have to remove your glucose monitor and insulin pump," another surgeon said.

I nodded, amazed by the flurry of activity around me. This was really happening.

"Your surgeon will be here in a moment," he said.

It was a moment I will never forget. Amidst the sea of scrubs and tubes emerged a familiar face through the doorway.

"Where's Boone?" the soft-spoken woman with the Minnesotan accent asked.

"He's with my roommate," I almost stammered. "Are you my surgeon?"

"Yes, I am," she replied.

What happened next is hard to describe. Tidal waves of relief washed over me. I felt my entire body relax and 30 years of tension simply vanished from my muscles. My eyelids grew heavy as tears began to collect under my eyelids.

"Everything looks good. The blood type and HLA are an identical match. We just got the organ, and I'm going to double check that everything is going to work out. But, I think we're good to go and you're going to have a Christmas worth remembering. We'll bring you back for surgery in about five minutes," she told me, in her kind, sweet, knowledgeable, confident voice.

The tears broke loose and ran down my face. This was the surgeon who got me. She saw me from the beginning. She gave me the facts. She understood my condition and she restored my faith in the healthcare system that I trusted my life to. I never imagined it would be her to perform this surgery but at that moment, I couldn't believe how fortunate I was. This was real. This was happening. And I had someone I trusted to see me through it.

My mom texted me to let me know she was on her flight. I sent her one message back, "It's a go. Putting my phone away. Let you know what's up when I can." I didn't know anything else, but that everything was a go. That's all I could say.

"Okay, here we go," the operating room nurse said as she began to wheel me back. "Oh, wait. I forgot to ask. Would you like to meet with the chaplain before we bring you back for surgery?"

"Yes," I said right away.

The chaplain was waiting outside the room and heard his cue to come in. He entered my room, with a gentle smile on his face. Everyone around me cleared out. Once we were alone, he asked if we could pray.

"Yes, please," I responded.

He prayed for the surgeons and transplant team and gave thanks to the donor whose pancreas would soon become mine. We prayed for the donor's family, as they were likely going through the exact opposite gamut of emotions that I was. The chaplain was quick and to the point, putting everything into perspective for me in a way I needed. He grounded me, as I was about to experience the most life changing event that could ever happen. At that moment I realized what was actually happening. Even with this realization, I simply couldn't believe it all.

"Okay, Brandon. Are you ready?" asked a nurse who was standing in the doorway with the surgeon's assistant.

"YES!"

As I was being wheeled into the operating room, I saw my surgeon along with two other surgeons standing around a stainless steel bowl. The pancreas was nestled inside. They were squirting liquid on it, using tools to get it ready for surgery, and monitoring it. Behind them, affixed to the wall, sat a huge whiteboard with my name and blood type on it. My X-rays and scans were hanging around the room, almost like posters in a teenager's bedroom. Everyone was so kind and courteous to me. I felt like I was in the right place and best of all, I felt comfortable. Was this actually happening?

"We have your mom's information and will be texting her updates until she arrives," a nurse informed me. I thanked her. *Perfect, I won't have to worry about that, and my mom will be kept in the loop*, I thought while laying there.

The anesthesiologist was in a different operating room helping another patient, someone told me. So a nurse moved me over to the other bed as they wheeled out the gurney. She got me in the right positions and put the oxygen mask on me all while trying to make conversation to pass the time. I looked around, taking everything in. At that moment I realized exactly what was going on. Granted, I knew there was always a chance that something could go wrong, but this was as close to getting a second chance at life as I would get. I made it.

"Here comes your anesthesiologist," the nurse said. I looked up at the kind faces above me, just thankful to be alive and to be able to receive this precious gift.

"Are you ready to start your new life?" the anesthesiologist asked me. I couldn't respond. I just nodded. Tears started rolling down my face, again, from the realization of all that had happened and was happening. I was full of gratitude. Then everything went black.

*   *   *

When I woke up, I knew immediately that this surgery was unlike any of my previous surgeries. There were no other patients in the recovery area. I had it all to myself. I blinked a few times before realizing someone was touching my side. I looked over and saw a nurse poking me gently, examining my wound.

"Hi," I said.

"Hi," she replied.

"Did it work?" I asked.

"Everything was successful," she responded with a smile.

It had happened. I survived. I had a pancreas transplant. I honestly expected to learn that the pancreas wasn't the perfect match, or there was some complication in surgery, or I needed a second kidney after all. I couldn't believe it. I felt amazing. Later, I learned that the surgery took four hours and recovery took about seven hours. I had tons of IVs sticking out of my arms and even my neck. I could press a button to administer medication whenever the pain emerged. The nurses were drawing my blood around the clock and testing my blood glucose levels. It kept coming back in the 80's.

It actually worked.

Once I saw that happen a few times, I knew I was going to be okay. I wanted to stay awake to see my mom and to monitor my new pancreas' progress, however my medical team urged me to go back to sleep.

"We're just checking for internal bleeding," they told me. "If we poke you, don't be alarmed."

They were going to transfer me from the surgical step-down unit to the ICU but didn't have any vacant beds available on the unit. It looked like I'd be staying in the recovery area for the time being. I went back to sleep.

Around 7:00 a.m., they finally were ready to move me to the

ICU. Several nurses hovered around my bed. I felt a little groggy, but I still knew what had happened and what was going on around me. I turned to the nurse by my right and asked, "Does my mom know what is going on?"

She smiled, "Yes. We've been keeping her updated with text messages until she arrived this morning. I'll bring her in as soon as we get you settled."

Relieved, I laid there as my body gradually woke up. The nurses rolled me down hallways and into elevators. Then the nurses put me in a lifting device and moved me into the hospital bed. I couldn't really move around the bed yet due to my staples and IVs. A few minutes later my mom appeared at the door to my room.

"I can't believe it," she said. "I can't believe this actually happened."

"I can't believe it either, Mom!"

My mom updated the family as nurses came in and out every 30 minutes to check on my staples, internal bleeding, test my blood sugar, and make sure I was comfortable. They continued to test my blood sugar every 30 minutes for the first day. It felt like Russian roulette. It would come back 112, then 70, and then 95. I kept waiting for it to bottom out, but it never did. For the first time in my life, I was not on insulin and my blood sugar remained normal. I hadn't crashed in over 12 hours.

By now, nearly everyone who followed my medical plight knew I had the surgery. Calls, emails, texts, and messages were coming in from all over. Everyone wanted to make sure I was doing okay. It was humbling. People told me they put me on their church's prayer list or that they set an intention for my good health each day. I just could not believe so many people cared about me. Whenever I received a call or text, I always expected bad news or someone asking for a favor. This genuine concern for my wellbeing was new for me. It was something I had only experienced with my immediate family. For so long I purposely kept people out of my life. I kept them at arm's reach. I didn't divulge my weaknesses or secrets, fearing that something could be used against me. Now, having overcome my worst fear, I learned the value of letting people in. It felt good to be genuinely cared about.

In addition to the nurses and doctors who kept checking on me, various people who were a part of this entire journey also stopped by to see how I was doing. My coordinators checked in. Individuals who were a part of my consultation process said congratulations and hello. After the third congratulations, I asked why everyone was saying that. They said that it's great news, and everyone who has a successful transplant is congratulated at the opportunity it presents. Even Shawna from finance made a point to check in.

"I knew the moment you were listed you were going to get that pancreas soon," she told me. "I couldn't tell you, but I knew it."

"Thank you for everything," I told her in earnest.

"You're welcome. Brandon, since I had a feeling your surgery would be sooner rather than later, I postponed my vacation. You were one of the few people who paid cash. You paid upfront. You followed through with everything. I knew when we called you that there would be confusion about lack of insurance on your account. I did not want my vacation to interfere with that."

"You didn't have to do that Shawna, but I am so glad you did!"

"Me too. Almost all the transplants are done through insurance. You are the exception to the rule. I wanted to make sure everything went smoothly."

I laughed. I had been the exception to the rules my whole life.

"Are you ready to go traveling?" she asked with a huge smile.

"I'm so ready to get back to living my life."

Shawna wished me well and congratulated me again before getting back to work. I was moved beyond words by her kindness and generosity. She didn't treat her role at Mayo as a job. She was a true patient advocate who really cared about people. I was so lucky to have met her through this process.

The next day my surgeon came in for a post-operative exam. My mom was getting coffee, and it was just the two of us.

"Thank you so much," I said.

"You're welcome, Brandon. I was just doing my job. And congratulations."

I expected her to check on my wound or my vitals but instead she just stood there smiling, like we were old friends.

"I am so happy for you. Everything looks as it should. I don't expect you will have any major issues."

"Wow, that is so amazing to hear," I said in disbelief.

"You have a second chance at life that many people do not get. It's time for you to go live it. Make sure to do what makes you happy," she told me before leaving the room.

The words hit me hard. She was right. I had a new life to live.

EPILOGUE

I remained in the ICU for five days. Recovery took around six weeks and my mom was by my side through it all. I am no longer an insulin dependent type 1 diabetic. The pancreas transplant makes and regulates my insulin correctly.

Around the third week of recovery, I remember getting in the shower and all of the sudden my feet felt like they were on fire. Startled, I shut the water off and looked down at them. Then it hit me...my feet were feeling the warmth of the water! I don't know how long I didn't feel the warmth of water on my feet because being a lifelong diabetic had damaged the nerves. Somehow, my body was healing internally. I was shocked at what I had lost without ever realizing it. I can only imagine what else my body is healing because now it's working properly.

However, at the fifth week of my recovery I began to experience organ rejection. I was nervous. I wondered if my life would return to my pre-transplant state...full of blood sugar crashes and unknowns. I wondered what I did wrong. After all this time, I felt like a failure. Why was my body not accepting this new and lifesaving gift? These questions and feelings of guilt were overwhelming. However, the doctors acted like it was no big deal and a normal thing. I was sent to have heavy steroid infusions to calm the organ. It seemed to work. But, this was not my first bout of rejection.

It was a long recovery, full of learning new and surprising discoveries. For one, I have to take lifelong medication that is far more expensive than any of my diabetic supplies were. I am now on immunosuppressants with side effects that impact my daily life. For example, I have extreme muscle cramps, my limbs shake near the end of the day, my hair falls out, I have to run to the bathroom multiple times a day, I experience extreme bloating, it takes me three times longer than normal to heal from a simple scratch, and I will get skin cancer because my body cannot produce melanin without an immune system.

I have to be very careful about not getting sick. I wash my hands constantly, stay away from sick people when possible, wear a face mask in crowds, wash fruits and vegetables three times, and everything has to be cooked well done. With a lowered immune system, I am now susceptible to every bacteria, virus, and fungi because my body cannot fight it off. My short-term memory is hindered, which could be from the medication or even from possible brain damage from all my low blood sugars before surgery. Today, I have more blood draws and doctor appointments than ever before. This is a small sacrifice to pay over being a type 1 brittle hypoglycemia unaware diabetic living in fear of fading away and never waking up.

Epilogue

I didn't wake up from surgery as a "perfectly fine" person who was magically cured of all ailments. The point of all of this, the surgery, the follow-up appointments, the medications, is to keep me healthy. I was a diabetic for 31 years and other complications come from that. They didn't go away. My transplant is simply a pause from what I was going through as a diabetic. The crazy part is, this transplant can last for the rest of my life or decide to reject my body tomorrow. Despite this, the hope is that things calm down in my body over time.

But I get to live each day, just a bit differently than if someone waved a wand and I was magically 100% cured. I am beyond grateful. It's amazing what can be done, really. I haven't had deadly low blood sugars or needed insulin since the transplant.

I was told to eat often and as much as I could. Unfortunately, the medication I was on took away my appetite; but when I could eat, I felt energized, the way it was supposed to be.

Diabetes taught me discipline and how to be a survivor. Having too much to eat at lunch would cause a high blood sugar that needed to be corrected. Correcting the high blood sugar generally would lead to a low blood sugar. It's a delicate balance. Even if you eat the same thing every day at the same time and give the appropriate amount of insulin each day and at the right time, it will rarely give you a duplicate day. Something is always off. So, you just have to learn how to roll with the diabetic life. Monitoring, counting carbohydrates, calculating insulin, injection, finger sticks, CGM and pump issues, batteries running low, insulin leaking, tube getting pulled, and mental fatigue.

I am still finding out what it's like to not have these thoughts in the back of my mind at all times. Eating without taking insulin is still taking time for me to understand. I have mental clarity, really for the first time. It's amazing what I can remember. It makes me wonder what life would have been like without diabetes. Although I didn't like others to know I had diabetes, I didn't feel like it held me back. I am excited to see what this "new life" has for me to experience.

This entire experience dramatically changed my whole perspective on life. Everything happened as it was supposed to. For many years, I lived this life where I swore I would never be a victim. I refused to let anything get in the way of my goals, only to become a victim and have to ask for help. Having to admit that I was vulnerable was the most difficult and greatest thing I have ever done. My hard and negative opinions of people, fostered by years of unfair experiences, gradually dissipated.

Numerous times I faced the impossible. I somehow worked through it. I was spared for a reason, perhaps so I could share my story and inspire others. Maybe it was to teach me the valuable lesson of letting people in or to finally be vulnerable. Whatever the case, I do not take my life saving surgery for granted. I beat the odds. No matter what each day brings, I'm just excited and so grateful that I'm able to experience it: good or bad. With one kidney, two pancreases, and 31 years with diabetes, I can truly say that I am the happiest that I have ever been. Everything that has happened led me to a place in my life that allows me to have the feeling of being free. Free from others' expectations of me. Free from being brought down by family, society, and my own expectations, and free to just embrace each day and live it to the fullest. I may have nothing to my name, but I have life and breath in my lungs.

Today, I'm alive. I invest my time in what I enjoy doing: bringing awareness to Diabetes and Chronic Illness because I couldn't find someone who had gone through what I was going through. I would have liked to ask questions but didn't have an opportunity and had to find everything out on my own. That is what inspired me to share my journey. Showing that life isn't always unfair or bad. Anything can happen. Boone has earned a much-deserved rest and enjoys spending his days relishing my company instead of trying to save my life. He still smells the air and walks up to me to smell my breath to see if I have a low blood sugar. It is amazing what dogs are capable of. Organ rejection is a very possible threat, so I need to be careful about stress and illness, but I have plans to share my story, since I get to remain on this earth a while longer.

People surprised me. Changed me. It showed me not to underestimate or overestimate others. I realized that in order to live life to the fullest, I had to learn forgiveness. I could not continue to let the past hold on to me. I'm not forgetting where I came from, but I am also not neglecting reaching for where I want to go. Each night when I go to sleep, I no longer worry whether I'll wake up. If I wake up, it's another day to enjoy, see everything this beautiful world has to offer, gain new experiences, learn, laugh, and not be bitter, angry, hurt, or sad. Life is simply too short to dwell on anything that is not going to add to my life. Every day is a gift and an absolute treasure.

Now, this isn't to say that everything in my life is now perfect. But I will say my opinion about life and the people in it has changed. I'm focused on being happy and making sure that moments, days, and opportunities are not taken for granted. We have so little time in this world and time is a gift we shouldn't waste. You have to use it while you have it. I thought I had it, then I lost it, but now I have it back. It took that loss for me to realize how precious time and life really are.

My purpose now is to motivate people to live their best life because everyone is suffering and struggling in some different way. I want to share my story so people know that they are not alone in this struggle against life, disease, family feud, mental illness, and whatever else is thrown at you. Even if everyone in your life has abandoned you, it doesn't mean you are alone—people change and can surprise you. Things are not always as they appear to be, and people can still be redeemed.

This entire journey has been strange and unique, but we all are strange and unique in our own ways. There are times for success and times for failure. I've learned to always self-advocate, no matter the circumstance. Cherish the smallest victory, for it is a victory, regardless. Kindness is one of the most powerful things humanity has to offer. And, as long as you're willing to fight despite insurmountable odds, you may just surprise yourself when you come out on the other side. Conquer your fear, stay resolute to your purpose, and do everything you can to make the most of the time you have. Whatever it takes to keep on kickin'.

AFTERWORD

Paula M. DeMore

*"You don't have a right to the cards you believe
you should have been dealt. You have an obligation
to play the hell out of the ones you're holding."*

-Cheryl Strayed, Tiny Beautiful Things:
Advice on Love and Life from Dear Sugar

A s a therapist, I often pass along this quote to my clients. Life goes sideways for us in so many different ways. Our suffering is what unites us as humans. It is not the exception; it is the rule. The prerequisite for our healing is acceptance, vulnerability, forgiveness. When I met Brandon, he was struggling with these concepts. Brandon presented as what we refer to in the therapy realm as "well defended." Life had taught him to protect himself, to close himself away from the understanding of others. He had watched his idyllic childhood disintegrate, saw the vagaries of mental illness overtake his father, and then experienced the abandonment of others who should have cared. He and his family had been betrayed by friends and extended family, the very people who should have supported them.

In response to his early traumatic injury, Brandon created a narrative in his mind to prevent further emotional harm, along with an edict: Don't emote, don't trust, don't let others in. Although this strict self-sufficiency may have been adaptive in the moment to mitigate his pain and make him feel more safe, this rule proved to be the antithesis of the belief system he would need to adopt to live as a young adult battling for his life. Brandon's attitude may have been what the Mayo social worker sensed when she mandated CBT therapy to qualify him for a transplant. I understood Brandon's frustration with the social worker's decision. I also knew he would need to shift his mindset in order to successfully navigate the path ahead. He would need to learn to trust, to assume the best about others, to ask for and accept help.

I introduced Brandon to Victor Frankl's conviction that we are in charge of our own stories. While we cannot control much of what befalls us during our lives, we alone get to decide how we will respond to these events: "Everything can be taken from a man but one thing: the last of the human freedoms—to choose one's attitude in any given set of circumstances, to choose one's own way." Viktor E. Frankl, *Man's Search for Meaning*. And so, through our work together, Brandon committed to letting down his guard, endeavoring to believe that people are doing their best, and beginning to trust that others' reactions to him were never about him. Another's unkindness or failure to support us is never about us; it is about that person's history, experience and flawed narrative. Others' reactions to us should not be taken personally; they simply have nothing to do with us. Brandon's situation was dire, life or death. He could control almost nothing, but he took charge of how he would react. Brandon played the hell out of the hand he was holding. Through his insight, strength and tenacity, Brandon beat the odds and is an inspiration to all of us struggling to be human in a sea of vulnerability.

This book is dedicated to the selfless hero who is my organ donor.

To my readers,

Please consider registering
to be an organ donor.

Made in the USA
Middletown, DE
07 August 2021

45590795R00118